I dedicate this book to my three daughters – Sophie, Emily and Chloe. Live good habits girls, celebrate life fully and love yourselves from the inside out. You are my greatest pride and inspiration.

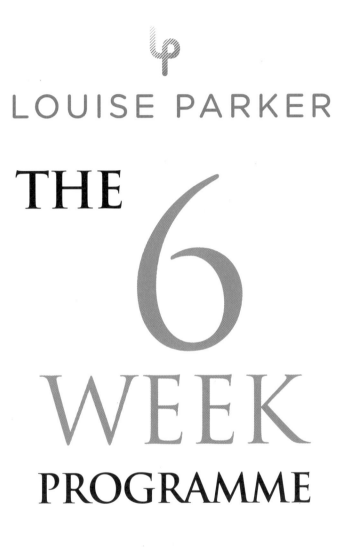

LOUISE PARKER

# THE
# 6
# WEEK
# PROGRAMME

Reshape your body
and change your
habits for life

MITCHELL BEAZLEY

I'm about to guide you through the first six weeks of a lifestyle overhaul, where you make yourself a priority and where your new habits will set you free.

# CONTENTS

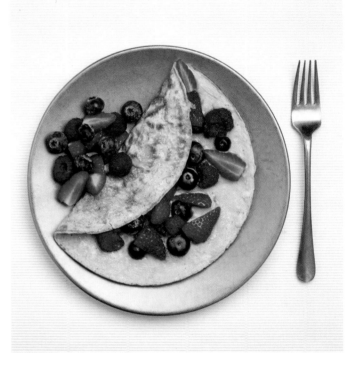

# INTRODUCTION

Have you ever wished you could press a reset button and lean towards a life of great habits and health? Why do some people just naturally maintain a healthy body and weight, and also seem to be the person at the table enjoying themselves and not engaging in 'diet chat'? I believe anyone can reset their habits, no matter what their history, age or obstacles. This book is for anyone truly wanting to change the way they live, reclaim their health and in doing so discover a body that's lean and strong and sustained with ease. It's about being the best version of yourself, being confident and happy in your skin and absolutely loving the way you live.

I created the Louise Parker Method for people just like me. It is such a joy to be free from the self-obsession of dieting and deprivation, and I'm so delighted that I have regained my life (and finally a body I feel really comfortable in, with its imperfections). My personal recovery story started where yet another failure ended. I just made up my mind that I would get off this tedious rollercoaster and stop punishing myself with the humungous effort involved in every quick-fix plan, all of which were totally unsustainable and therefore a complete waste of time, tantrums and tears.

I suspect, like most clients who come to us, your initial motivation for reading this book is 'I just want to lose this (grabs stomach, bum, backs of arms)' or perhaps you are saying to yourself 'I've tried everything, and it's just time to do it properly now'. However, I think we all know that the only way to achieve a permanent aesthetic result which thrills you, or to totally awaken your energy levels and motivation in all aspects of life, is to make a lifestyle shift. This can be an overwhelming thought as we are totally bombarded with conflicting information and we don't know where to start. It's all too tempting to think

'I'll just try this latest (insert current fad diet trend) to drop a dress size first; then I'll change my lifestyle'. You're focusing on the prize and not the process. I believe you've got to keep your eye firmly on that prize (and it has to be so much more than a size, number or weight – you deserve to be fit, happy and free) but the process has to become the focus. The process will become your habits. Your habits will take over and then you won't have to focus on the process.

And that's the sweet spot. I never bore of clients waxing lyrical about their body transformations, and my amazing team being so delighted in a client's result. But what trumps it all, is when we hear 'It's just so easy – I can't be doing it right', 'It makes total sense – I just wish I'd found you guys years ago – I'd have saved myself so much time and effort' or 'I'll never go back – why would I? – I love it, the Method's a pleasure and just how I live now'. When we refer to a client's success, it's actually more often in saying 'They've got it', rather than quoting a number on a scale.

Think of the *Louise Parker: The 6 Week Programme* as a lifestyle reset. Of course you're going to get beautiful results – but the purpose is to really inspire you and help you consistently touch base with each pillar of our Method long enough for the habits of health to kick in. You might get a bikini body in six weeks, but I urge you not to make that your focus. Focus on acquiring the habits. Habits are the key to long-term success and are what will almost effortlessly keep you in that sweet spot of health and freedom.

You have to change your mindset to believe that, from today onwards, the programme you are about to begin will become the foundation of how you will live.

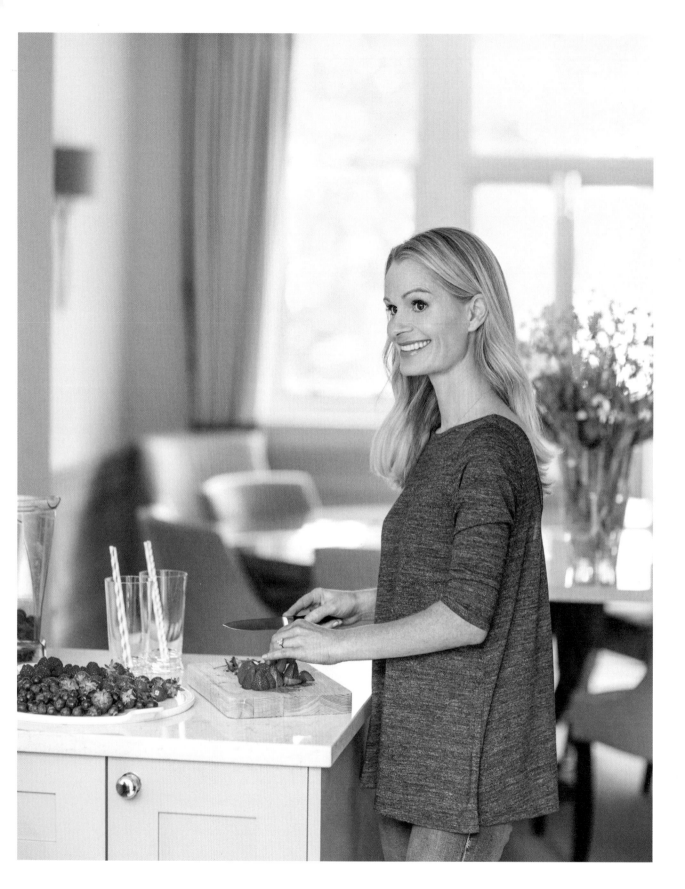

# WHY I WROTE THIS BOOK

I have a mission to end dieting and it's important to keep stating it. As I said in my first two books, by the time my three daughters are grown up, I'd like them to think dieting is as absurd as smoking was on planes, not so very long ago. I hope that, when I confess I did both, they'll be horrified. This is not a diet book and the Louise Parker Method is not a 'diet'. The idea is simply to reset how you eat, until it becomes a habit that you sustain, most of the time, once you're in a body you're chuffed with.

Since its inception, the fundamentals of the Louise Parker Method have not changed. The basic science is still the science and the core principles remain at the core. We have developed as a team and refined the way in which we coach our clients to reflect new research and developments – mainly the growing importance of sleep, mindfulness and the power of mindset on the path to success.

My first book – *The Louise Parker Method: Lean for Life* – explained the Method in detail and was so well received by so many of you – thank you. I gave you as much as I could pack into my first book, but you were left to navigate yourself through each week. My second book – *Lean for Life: The Cookbook* – summed up the Method and gave you over 140 recipes to keep you inspired and eating beautifully (sometimes simply and sometimes with a bit more effort for party days and celebrations but really, it's fit, fast food). The more you practise our style of eating, the quicker it becomes.

I'm hoping you bought this third book because you were inspired by my first two and are eager for more content and continued motivation. And because you want to genuinely change your lifestyle and learn to manage your weight once and for all.

Perhaps this is the first Louise Parker book you have – in which case, welcome aboard – you're intrigued to try a new approach to managing your health and it's come just at the right time. Perhaps like many of our clients, you're just utterly perplexed and bombarded with too much information and you don't know where to begin. Maybe you feel you actually invest as much precious time and effort into your body as you can – but you're demotivated and frustrated that you're not getting the return on your investment. We all tend to feel a bit hard done by in the results department – but I promise you that if you commit to our Method, make yourself accountable and, most of all, activate that consistency button for the first six weeks – you'll be winning. That means taking a leap of faith – leaving aside your doubts or concerns about your metabolism and your age and anything you're using as an excuse to stop you actually starting – and allowing me to guide you through the Method, week by week.

I'll continue to remind you of the importance of lifestyle and mindset in a world where we tend to look solely at calories in and calories out. There's so much more to it – but to keep it as simple and easily digestible as possible, I'm breaking it into bite-sized actions each week and points to gently guide you into taking better care of yourself. So, whether you've slipped a little or a lot, your motivation constantly wobbles or you've been told you're in danger of developing diabetes and really need to take stock – this programme is for you.

> To keep it as simple and easily digestible as possible, I'm breaking it into bite-sized actions each week and points to gently guide you into taking better care of yourself

# THE PURPOSE OF
# THE PROGRAMME

The purpose of this six-week programme is twofold:

Firstly, to offer those of you who already follow the Method some extra content – further delicious recipes so that you can keep ringing the changes, and some fresh, progressive workouts to support your metabolism, mobility and posture.

Secondly, to guide all of you through each of the pillars that make up the Method, one week at a time. I'm going to refresh you on them shortly, and even if you're a follower, do read the information again as the more positive brainwashing, the better. Each week I am going to give you tips and tasks, reminders and motivation – and generally cheer you along as I would a client of ours or a friend – to get you to the finish line of your 42-day reset. By the end of it, you'll be feeling fantastic, have renewed discipline and habits and really truly understand that there is no finish line. You won't actually want there to be.

I'm also going to refresh you on 'the dance' and the balance – because making the Method a part of you is absolutely fundamental to your long-term success.

I've kept true to my 'fit, fast food' approach to recipes and have tried to give you a good mix – some speedier, some more suitable for batch-cooking and taking to work, some that lend themselves to days you want to make an effort. After I'd written the recipes, I realized that, actually quite accidently, over 50 per cent were vegetarian or vegan. I suppose I've gradually developed more of a plant-based diet for myself and my family and, while I still love a bacon buttie, I guess this natural lean towards a more 'flexitarian' way of eating is reflected in the recipes. I naturally chose to share my recent recipes with you from my kitchen to yours.

Workout wise, there's more material to motivate you each week and I'm going to take you through what I'd like you to aim for. The workouts are both harder and simpler than those in the first book, sequenced and progressive. I've kept the focus on getting the best bang for your buck out of your time investment. It's effective.

I've maintained the balance of mindset reminders, inspiration and tips and tricks with the first and second pillars of the Method: Think Successfully and Live Well. I hope that these pillars really keep you inspired as the weeks go by, and they prompt you on days that perhaps the flesh is willing but the mind is weak, or the other way round. Don't neglect them as 'fluff'. You have to make yourself a priority and feel passionate in order to achieve the lasting results you long for.

Yes, there's a time promise – because we all need a period of time to get rid of inertia and allow the healthy habits to take hold. And in this time, as a side-effect of the changes you are about to make, you'll discover a body that swiftly changes into a much healthier, tighter, fitter, beautifully nourished version of what it is today.

Once the pillars all start working together and have you firing on all cylinders, you won't mind if you have to do another 42 days. The idea is that you'll be happy to follow my Method for another 42 years (actually living it *most* of the time and learning the art of balance the rest of the time, so you can eat cake and drink cocktails and not become a health bore).

So I'm not adding any new gimmicks or gizmos in this book, but focusing on what I hope you will find to be refreshing and inspiring new content. I'm about to guide you through the first six weeks of a lifestyle overhaul, where you make yourself a priority and where your new habits will set you free.

# HOW CHANGING MY MIND CHANGED MY BODY

The Louise Parker Method is now 22 years old. I've spent half my life dedicated to it. During the first ten years, I devised my first six-week programme and taught it personally to hundreds of clients. As a personal trainer, I combined four exercise sessions per week, each 90 minutes, with a complete dietary overhaul. I devised my Method by literally sitting down one day and jotting it on a piece of blue paper in about an hour. I remember it like it was yesterday.

It was the culmination of every book and article known to man that I'd digested – or not digested – combined with hundreds of case studies from my life as a trainer, and a sort of awakening through all the lessons I'd learned from all the mishaps and misery I'd endured starting and stopping so many unobtainable, promise-led diet plans. I simply wanted a balanced, sociable life and a perkier arse.

I actually wrote it for myself in a moment of desperation as I'd been on and off the diet treadmill since I was 14 years old. I was sick and tired of being sick and tired, losing and gaining the same ten or twenty pounds for a decade. That's a lot of wasted time, money and energy. I was just so fed up with failing and defining myself by my latest fad and what I looked like, not what I actually felt like. It led me to rock bottom and from there I knew that it was time to do it properly, kindly and sensibly.

I wish I knew then what I know now. That losing weight, toning your body, having the energy to lean into life and truly embrace it shouldn't be painful. And that if you're consistent and smart, it won't take long either. It has to become part of you, not something that you are 'doing'. Stop squeezing so tightly, find a zone in which there is pleasure and it becomes a permanent life change.

It is about getting your head down for a while as you truly acquire the habits of the Method – and then the lifestyle balance kicks in. You need a certain amount of time for this to kick in and become part of you. It will require a bit of mental toughness and a positive mental attitude and I'm going to help week by week with thoughts and tips and tasks that have helped me. Sometimes there will be things that you don't feel like doing but I know that this discipline can be learned – and before you know it, the habits will kick in. Don't underestimate what you can achieve in terms of a lifestyle reset in six weeks.

Practise the Method for long enough – beyond this 42-day reset – and it will just feel like breathing. Every now and again you'll hiccup, but you'll go back to breathing again afterwards. You're never going to feel guilt over a hiccup.

No matter what your age or how many times you have tried to change, please believe me when I say that it is never too late to start over. If you aren't fulfilled with your lifestyle, try something different – something that has worked for thousands of others before you, from every single age group and some with the most astounding challenges in life. The next six weeks are going to pass anyway – let's just get started.

It's worked for me and changed my life for the better in every single way. I believe we're all forever a work in progress, and that's how it should be. I'm far from the finished article and love the idea that I'm continually evolving. I don't feel bouncy every day and there are weeks when working my hardest, raising three young children (albeit with an amazing husband who more than pulls his weight) leaves me bone tired and wanting to nap for a month. But I've learned that I have to put my health and habits first if I'm going to be fully prepared for everything in my life that's so important to me. In order to do more and be more, I have to do less and care for myself first. If not, it can all unravel and everyone suffers.

Simply put, I make my habits my priority. I, too, have to reset them every now and again and in doing so I'm healthy and happy and I've got more confidence and contentment in my forties than I did in my twenties. Which is ultimately what we all deserve: to be able to live our best life. I'm actually excited about my sixties and motivated by my clients who are nearly twenty years older than me.

# LOUISE PARKER METHOD – THE BASICS

I want to outline the basics for you before we set everything in motion. It's important to grasp the principles so you know that each small action you take is key to taking you a step closer to the habit breakthrough. Every positive action connects to another and you'll soon find that practising and repeating all four pillars in conjunction with each other makes the whole journey easier. The more pillars you weave into your routine on a daily basis, the more stability you give to the process as your body actually works with you to make it easier. If you're motivated and determined, take regular rest and sleep, your mood and hormones behave in a way that allows you to actually want to reach for foods that fuel you, and it becomes so much more natural to throw on your trainers. It's all interconnected. Each pillar helps the others and they work together to make the journey easy, effective and a forever solution.

The Louise Parker Method is not a six-week celebrity, beach body, magical 'diet'. You may not get a beach body in 42 days – but you'll be well on your way. It's a fat loss and lifestyle overhaul and if you practise it reliably, one day at a time (as best you can – forgiving yourself when you hiccup), the four pillars will rally together to actually help your motivation and habits stick. They're in it together to help you. It will become a way of life that I passionately believe to be the simplest, sanest and healthiest solution to a healthier life – and an impressive body transformation.

Ultimately, you have to put the work in, make the commitment, and your results are going to match the consistency of your actions. What you put in, you will get out. If you dabble with a couple of pillars and obsess over one or two, you won't get the ultimate result and you won't find it as easy as you should. Just don't be mediocre about it. What you do every day will define your future self.

It's really an attitude. Our thoughts dictate our actions and commitment. And your actions are going to dictate your result and the longevity of it. Your results are going to dictate how you feel, and firm up a great attitude – and

once you're in this circle of success, you'll pull yourself round and round and round.

So – think of it as a style of living which blends eating beautifully, working out intelligently, embracing a positive mindset and making some simple lifestyle changes. It's a real-life solution for optimum health and well-being. Once you're ready to go into the Lifestyle Phase, you'll still have all the 'worth it' pleasures of life and celebration, in beautiful balance. No more yo-yo diets and deprivation. You're still going to eat roast potatoes and let your hair down at parties – we're just delaying that for a little while, while you get into the habit of how you're going to live most of the time.

The next 42 days are the beginning of your habit makeover and the end of self-obsession, yo-yo dieting and sabotaging all that is good for you. Please, please focus on the habit and the results will look after themselves.

I think the ultimate health and happiness prescription for anyone is to find a routine that they love and just happens to be really damn good for them.

## THREE PHASES = TRANSFORM, BALANCE, LIFESTYLE

At Louise Parker we coach the Method in three phases – Transform (what you're about to embark on), Balance and Lifestyle. Our clients may do one or two rounds of our six-week Transform programme, followed by Balance, where we coach them to start incorporating risotto and Rioja and all their 'worth its' into life, until living in balance just becomes a habit too. Then in the Lifestyle Phase, we see them once a month to make sure that they remain on track, that the habits are really consolidating naturally and provide a good tweak and accountability check. Many clients complete the 6–12-week Transform, while others do a year-long programme, where they reach their goal perhaps after four or five months and we spend the remaining time coaching the Lifestyle Phase, training that habit so strong, it's set for life.

# THE FOUR PILLARS OF THE LOUISE PARKER METHOD

The Method is about immersing you in all pillars of the programme long enough for everything to feel like what I like to call your New Normal. But even while you're waiting for that magical moment to kick in, please try to focus on just paying some attention to each pillar, every day. One day at a time, that's all. Think of getting your head on your pillow every night having done your damn well best, and don't project about how much weight you want to have lost in 21 days. Those who focus on the habits and not the result have a speedier, less turbulent ride and arrive at a much sunnier place. I WOULD YELL THIS IF I COULD. I think it is the key to success and longevity of results.

## 1. THINK SUCCESSFULLY

- Practise a strong mental attitude and 'can-do' approach. A strong mental attitude and an absolutely-bloody-well-can-do approach is essential to the success of everything in life and this re-programme is no exception. What you want out of it, you're going to have to put in.

- Visualize your New Normal in technicolour and assume that you are going to follow it through and just nail it. Forget every past diet that you've rebounded from. It wasn't sustainable and so failed you – you are not the failure. You need a vision that's so clear to you that it can motivate you through the toughest of days. And you're going to need this vision to prop up your motivation, until the habits kick in. Your vision has to be bold, it has to be enticing or it's just not going to propel you forward on the days when you need that boost. We'll really look at this in your Prep Week.

- Practise mental toughness on days that challenge you until a natural discipline falls into place. We do have to work at motivation – it requires a mental power and eventually your brain (just like a muscle) will get stronger, the longer you practise replacing your doubtful thoughts with optimism and determination. Don't think it's a given for anyone – it's tough to start but vastly simpler to sustain once up and running.

- Make yourself an absolute priority and be accountable. Learn to carve out some time to put yourself first. There will be days when you are being yanked left, right and centre, and you may only be able to move an inch in the right direction – but to keep it moving is key. Do something for yourself every single day that's good for you. The alternative is that you burn out or throw the towel in and that's just not an option.

## 2. LIVE WELL

- Take great pride and pleasure in your surroundings and self – it has such a profound effect on your mindset and mood, which positively spill over into every area of your new lifestyle.

- Dedicate yourself to 'digitally detoxing' from screens and really commit to a pampering bedtime routine. Regular sleep is the simplest way to make huge strides in everything we do. It's the foundation of your health.

- Make a conscious effort to rest when you can and diminish stress in a world where we are constantly being bombarded – a calmer routine is going to make for a much more relaxed reset.

- Really take time to stop, notice and adjust your weekly routine so that you're constantly moving towards a lifestyle that you take huge pleasure in and in which you operate at your best.

## 3. EAT BEAUTIFULLY

- You'll eat in balance – a little protein, a little good fat and a good dose of low-GI carbs at every meal, and space it out – a dietician-approved method that works and is totally fad free. The eating habits you lean into over the reset are going to become the foundation of how you eat forever.

- You're going to hydrate yourself well and cut out booze and sugar for the reset. They're not banned forever, but they will slow down the setting of concrete habits.

- Make a pact to prepare meals that you actually love, that your friends and family can enjoy too. Really be open minded to making your meals a pleasure – and take pride in how you present them to yourself. Find the delicious and bin the 'diet food' menu.

- Practise eating well on the go, on the run and while eating out. You cannot put your life on hold while you set your new habits – learning to eat as best as you can in any situation is imperative. It's not a plan I want you to lock yourself away for – it's a real-life solution so we're going to end the start-and-stop mentality that so many dieters have. That will give you the greatest sense of freedom, I promise.

## 4. WORK OUT INTELLIGENTLY

- By committing in Week 1 to become an active person, someone who simply moves more daily, you will ease into an energetic life and wake up that part of you that actually wants to move. You will stop thinking about exercise as a burden. Keep an open mind about trying new activities and you'll soon wake up a body that was born to move – and watch how your life changes.

- You will have an at-home 'cardio-conditioning' routine to follow which changes fortnightly, to build a strong and mobile body, while burning through any excess body fat. The focus is on getting the best results possible for your time and once you're in the groove, you're going to slot quick, effective workouts into most days of your life.

- These workouts will progress and you'll soon start reaping the rewards of a stronger, leaner and more flexible body which burns more body fat at rest. Yup, in a few weeks you're actually going to speed up your metabolism as we preserve valuable muscle by eating and working out intelligently.

- You're going to take it a day at a time and put your absolute all into making an active lifestyle a pleasure and practise discipline to 'pay your daily rent' on the days that you find it a challenge. It's going to require you to dig deep some days but the trick is to just keep it moving. A strong body is only ever on loan – the rent is due every week.

# HOW TO USE THIS BOOK

The format of this book is very different from my first two. For the best results possible, pick up a copy of both my previous books and really get immersed. But all the basics are here.

## READ, LEARN, ABSORB

I'm going to talk you through the four pillars of my Method to highlight the importance of integrating them all into your lifestyle. Remember that it is a bit like a four-legged stool. If you're balanced on all four legs, you're in a super-stable place. On three, you'll probably stay upright, but with the odd wobble. Two and you're just making it harder for yourself. One and you're going to fall on your arse. It's the power of the pillars coming together that is the magic of the ease, results and sustainability of the Louise Parker Method.

## THE PREP WEEK

I'm then going to take you through a Prep Week (and I really want you to do this, to get organized, read up and really absorb all the information). Don't jump straight in – even with our coached programmes, we purposefully build in time between the initial consultation and kick-off before we start a client's journey – as there's information you just need to absorb and it's good to have time to get excited and truly behind it. This is not to be confused with a week where you go and have a total blowout. That would not be clever, just self-sabotage. In this week you're preparing to get into really positive headspace, making you good to go.

## READ IT ONCE, THEN READ IT AGAIN

As part of your Prep Week, I'd like you to read through the book once, and then read it again. If you can, familiarize yourself with my first book, *The Louise Parker Method: Lean for Life*. Make notes where you need to and jot down things that really resonate with you, maybe nuggets of information that hit a chord and you know that you

will have to focus on a little bit more. Keep it by your bed, snapshot pages which inspire you and keep them on your phone. Do whatever it takes to get behind your decision.

## SWAP AROUND, BE FLEXIBLE

I've purposefully written this guide to allow you to choose your own meals because one-size-fits-all menu plans are frustrating and because I don't want you using the fact that you can't drink a chocolate smoothie on Day 23 at 11am as an excuse to say 'I'm sure it works for everyone else, but I travel and don't have a blender'. I encourage you to pick your own meals and snacks from any of my recipes and devise your own recipes once you've got the principles. It works whoever you are – full stop. The only exception is if you don't want it enough (but we're going to practise a can-do mindset). You can adapt your meals to suit your lifestyle, whether you're single and work a nine-to-five job, you have three kids and are looking after elderly parents, or you're someone who's constantly on the go with a really unpredictable life.

I'd love you to try to throw your all into it – like anything, the more you put into it, the more you will get out of it. You've total control over when to do your workouts and what recipes to eat on what days. I've made it as flexible as possible. Please don't use barriers as an excuse, or at least recognize them for what they are. See the obstacles and leap over them.

## THE SIX WEEKS

Then I start taking you through your reset, week by week. Try to select the recipes that jump out at you (don't force yourself to eat anything you dislike – I want you to love your grub), choosing how much time you want to invest in the kitchen and what works for you and your family. This time round I've put all the main meals into one section so you can swap around supper and lunch (and do the same from books one and two). I've broken them down into suggestions for when they work but do feel free to mix these up and keep ringing the changes. There are heaps and heaps of options to choose from.

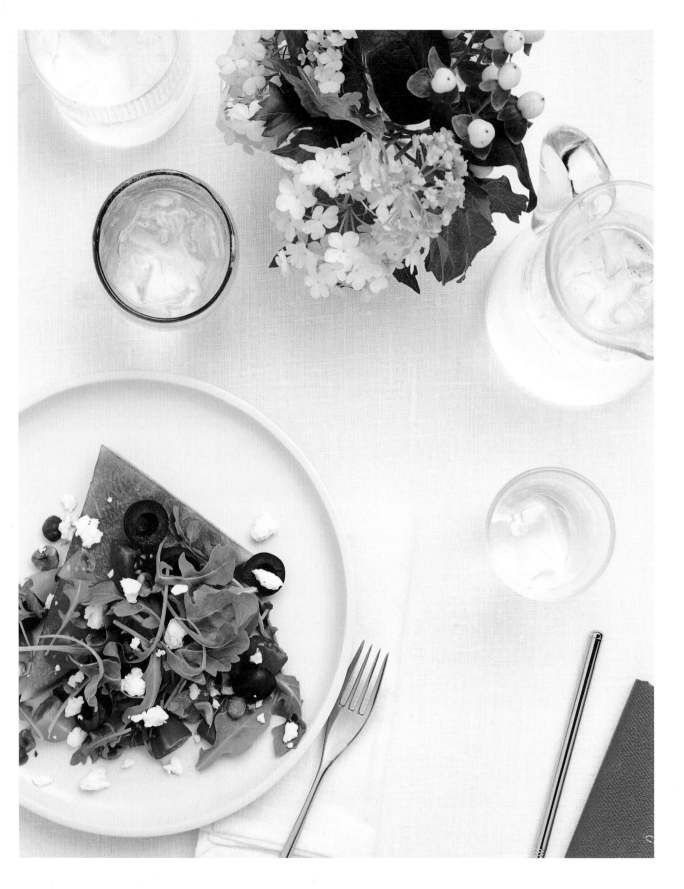

Every week, I'm going to talk you through your workouts and activity and give you little nuggets of motivation and some tasks to take on which I know will help your journey. You may wonder what clearing out your junk drawer has to do with your health – these are all optional pointers which help bring order to chaos on those days when we feel frazzled. You're going to take time out to rest, pamper and create a more peaceful life. And developing and really training yourself to practise a winning mindset and approach to your lifestyle is going to help set the happy habits. It may take some practice but, like anything, give it time and attention and you'll build strong habits. It's your mindset that will protect your results forever. Time to let go of doubt and fear of failure and look forward with steely determination.

## PROGRESSIVE WORKOUTS THAT CHANGE FORTNIGHTLY

For maximum results, I'm changing your workout schedule every fortnight. I'll take you through each fortnight and constantly challenge you. It's important to keep adapting your routine and you'll find that, as you tick off your workouts, you'll be ready to go onto the next step. Your body will adapt at a brilliant rate, but you've got to get the workouts in before you move onto the second and third workout regimes. Our bodies thrive on change and surprise – it forces them to adapt and strengthen, which is exactly what we want. So, as well as the home workouts becoming more challenging, you're going to increase your movement too – increasing your steps every week and then stepping out of your comfort zone and finding new physical challenges. The progression and adaptation are not only going to keep your muscles engaged and challenged, but keep your mind focused too. You're going to feel the most wonderful sense of achievement as you find your body capable of doing so much more than it does today, in as little as six weeks.

## REPEAT THE CYCLE – DON'T STOP UNTIL THE MAGIC HAPPENS

Please remember that this six-week programme is a kick-start. It's a RE-programme. Some of you are going to go straight to your goal, it'll be enough to get you to your best body, and the habits will just click into place. More of you will benefit from repeating the programme – remember that the programme is a Method, a way of life that never really ends. It simply loosens, you relax into celebrating when it's 'worth it' and in time you'll learn to live it almost intuitively, as I do now.

It may take you four weeks, it may take you four months – but habits worth having are worth the effort of acquiring. You'll get there in your own time and the more you seek the pleasure in those habits, the sooner they will set. The sooner they set, the sooner you get all the benefits that come with them.

Once you're at goal, you stick to those habits roughly 70–80 per cent of the time (depending on how active you are) and I promise it will set you free. No more dieting. No more 'last hurrah' or 'diet starts Monday' mental-ity. No more guilt over missing a workout, writing off food groups, searching for the magic answer. Remember, you're redesigning your lifestyle to one you enjoy more and reap endless benefits from, so you won't ever want that to end. You may want a glass of wine, but you can have it. And freshly baked bread with salty butter. Nothing is being taken away forever. But first we need to reset what you do MOST of the time (and align it with pleasure), then you continue to celebrate with the best of them SOME of the time.

It'll be so worth waiting for your Lifestyle Phase. By then you'll know what you actually find 'worth it' and it gives you the time to settle into a new way of doing things.

Later I'll share with you how I make the Lifestyle Phase work – my way of life. There's not one set rule and we adapt it for each client and help them navigate what works for them until it becomes intuitive. But it's simply about loosening the reins when you're celebrating and, crucially, giving up the 'on it' or 'oh bugger it' mentality. That's the biggie and where most people's weight fluctuation lies. Between those two phrases, not a Sunday lunch and Monday breakfast.

Once you get this, you have a blueprint for living and you'll never have to start or stop a fad again. How amazing would that be?

## TICK OFF THE WEEKS & THE TASKS

It sounds a bit school-like, I know, but I genuinely think we all respond well to tasks and there'll be a good sense of accountability (and hopefully pride) that will come from each little tick. Think of it as your own personal accountability check – not a test or anything you might fail at. It's all positive progress.

## BALANCE & LIFESTYLE

Once you've completed the six-week programme, you'll be well on your way to establishing fit, healthy habits for life. This is when we can start to introduce your 'worth its' and you'll intuitively judge when you do and don't want to step out of the circle. See pages 130–4 for more.

## WHEN TO START

We often say that the best time to do a Louise Parker programme is when your life is busy. My motto is 'Now is always a good time to begin'. Weddings, holidays and work trips shouldn't prevent you from starting a new lifestyle. Remember that this is a reset of your lifestyle

and not a six-week bootcamp. We find that when clients are coached throughout really busy periods of life, the results are even better. They may lose a pound less with challenges in their way, but the FOCUS is learning how to live the Method in real life, so I always see that as a positive. Alongside their results, they learn how to adjust the plan depending on what challenges are put in their way, and this is invaluable. I just love it when I hear a client say they've not only managed their first all-inclusive holiday on the Method, but have taken a step forward. Our lives are demanding and eventful and there will *never* be a chunk of time where everything simply stops.

You might not feel that this is the 'right time' for you. There never is a right time. We are never really ready, so all I would say is just start before you are ready. You will never have a six-week window where life pauses – and the key to long-term success is learning the moves of the Method while life's ups and downs are happening around you.

The beauty of the Method is that you can do it on the go, eating out, on flights and trains – you don't have to put your life on hold. I'll give you lots of tips on how to do this. Delaying starting because of a New Year's Eve weekend is an excuse to procrastinate. The sooner you start, the sooner you reach your destination, even if you have to step outside of the circle for an evening. I once read the following quote from the actor Hugh Laurie and keep it on my phone as it's always a great reminder to me if I'm procrastinating over something. It really strikes a chord with me. 'It's a terrible thing, I think, in life to wait until you are ready. I have this feeling now that no one is ever ready to do anything. There is almost no such thing as ready. There is only now. And you may as well do it now. Generally speaking, now is as good a time as any.'

## IT'S JUST A DANCE

If you are familiar with my first books, you will be familiar with this concept but it's one other thing I will repeat as I know it's something that literally hundreds of followers have written to me to say it really helped them get it. It made them learn the Balance and Lifestyle Phases and give up the 'all-or-nothing' mindset that plagues a dieter's mind.

Think of the Louise Parker Method as a dance which, when you learn the steps and practise them (the four pillars), will become part of who you are, your habits, something you just do and not a plan you are 'doing' for now. The habits are always with you.

Imagine an inner circle, which represents the core of the Method. You should aim to spend as much of your time as you can in this inner circle over the next 42 days (or longer if you decide to continue with the Transform Phase for longer). I'm suggesting staying as close as possible to the inner circle, because it will actually be quicker for you to achieve your goal and acquire those habits. You're not always going to be bang in the middle of that circle, but that's okay – you just strive to stay as close to it as you can.

Now imagine an outer circle. When you've reached your goal and switched to the Lifestyle Phase of the Method, you will probably spend 20–30 per cent of your time in the outer circle, depending on how active a lifestyle you live. It does vary and no calculators are needed. You step out of the inner circle when it's worth it (maybe a slice of birthday cake, a glass of wine on a Friday night), but then you step back in again, step out, step back in. However, you always come back to the inner circle again because that's where you live now. Sometimes you'll stay out a little longer – that's normal (Christmas, holidays, tricky times perhaps) but it just means you've got to balance it out with more time bang in the middle of the inner circle just as soon as you can. The main thing is that you always return home to the inner circle – and don't stray for too long, or it's just harder to come back to a place that you actually love living when you are there.

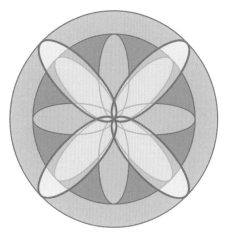

You're going to learn what is really 'worth it' to you, the things you feel are worth stepping out of the inner circle for. For me, it's meals out with my family a couple of times a week, a few glasses of wine spread across the week with my husband or girlfriends, baking with my girls or maybe a Mr Whippy in the park.

The point is, don't let Mr Whippy take you to the point of no return and say 'bugger it'. It's not a winning mindset to use eating something not on Method as a reason to say you've 'failed', 'cheated' or (God forbid) to call it a 'sin'. This is my biggest peeve and it's an excuse people use not to succeed. 'I've ruined the whole thing now' is an attitude that will keep you stuck in the past. A Mr Whippy is always just a Mr Whippy.

You'll naturally become really selective about what goes in your mouth – because you're so much more aware of what actually pleases you and what's not worth your while. It's a type of self respect that becomes so much more natural when you're generally living in the midst of the Method.

Just step straight back into the inner circle after you've stepped out – it genuinely is just a dance. Don't give up or think you've given in to eating any food that is a celebration or joy. Don't try to be perfect, because perfection is such an illusion. For now we are going to try to keep you bang in the middle of the circle as we have habits to set. But remember, if you step out – don't jump on a three-week bender – just step straight back in.

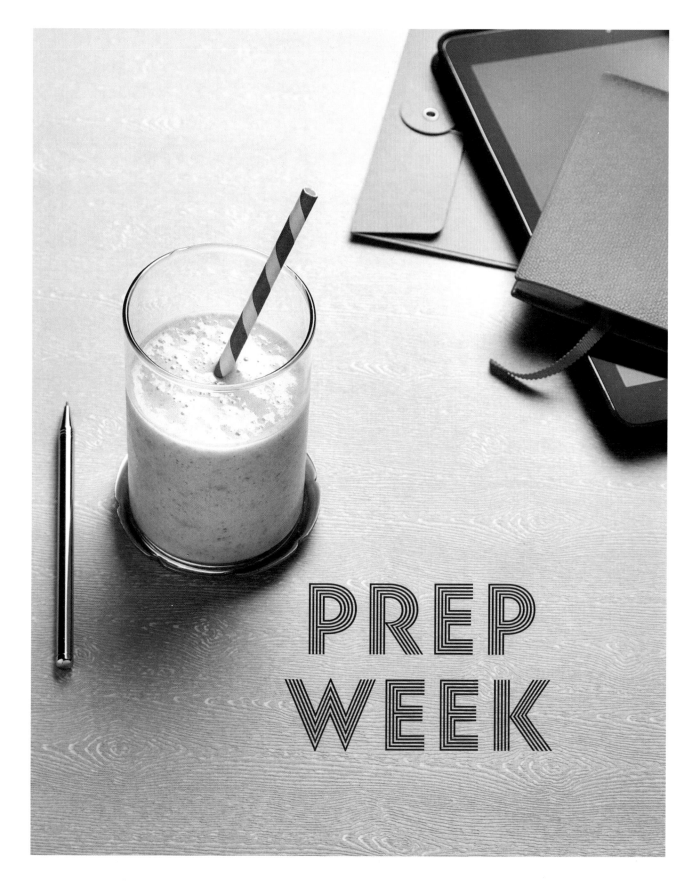

PREP
WEEK

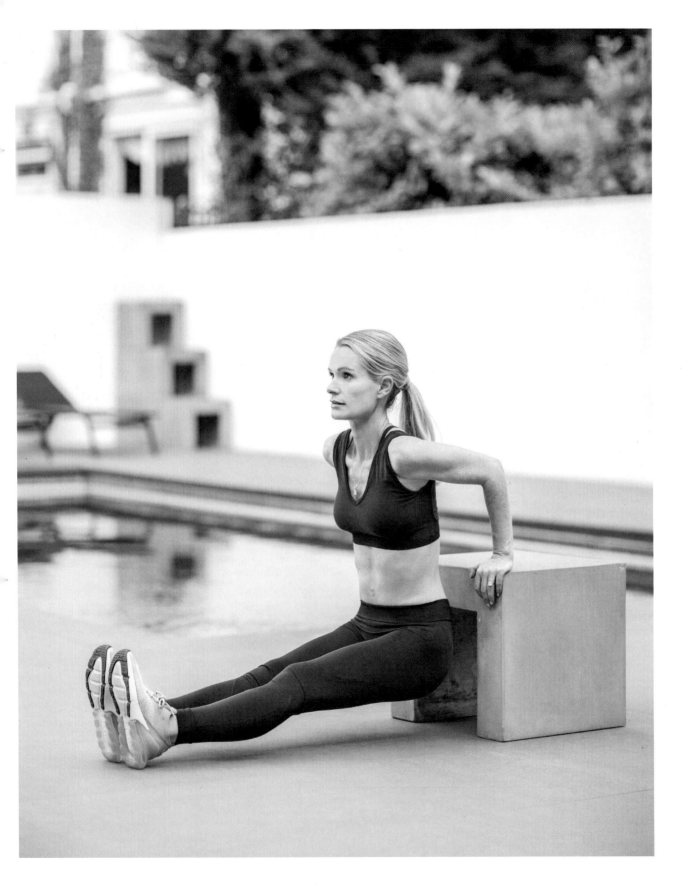

Even if you're absolutely raring to go, please take my advice and take a week to get prepared for your programme. It's one wee week to digest new information, get yourself in order and just have some time to reflect on what you can do to pave a clearer path. It's crucial to prepare – mentally and physically – for something that's going to be your focus for the next few weeks.

You're slowly easing into the Method this week, laying down some new routines so that you kick off Week 1 feeling ready, more rested and having jumped off the sugar train. The Prep Week is the foundation – you won't build stable habits on flimsy groundwork.

# PREPARING TO THINK SUCCESSFULLY

## 1. JUST KEEP IT OPEN

My very first bit of advice for your Prep Week is to keep an open mind. That's all. I'm so confident that if you throw your full commitment into the programme for six weeks, you're going to ignite confidence, not just in yourself, but in the Method. And you're going to be just thrilled with how straightforward it is, once you've got organized, understood the four pillars and just got into the groove of things. It's easy for me to say because I know it works.

The only barrier – and I'll say it again – is doubt. Doubt in something that will work for you as well as everyone else, doubt in your ability to see it through – when perhaps you've not achieved success in this area of your life before. I suspect you're really successful in countless other areas of your life and perhaps healthy habits are the missing link. Think of something that you've overcome and seen through to the end, even when it was tough. Right, you did that – and so you can do this. Don't see it

as a mountain to climb. Don't perceive it to be difficult – it isn't. It's as difficult as your head wants to make it. Every time a doubt pops into your head, just flick it off as you would an annoying fly. It's just feeding on your 'stinking thinking'. Every negative thought that pops in, tell it where to go, and replace it with something you'd say to motivate a friend.

I'm whacking this right up front, because learning to push away every downer of a thought takes persistence – until you feel yourself change – both mentally and physically. Have some faith in yourself – you can do anything for six weeks. Don't think beyond that for now. Have utter faith for a week or two if that's all you can manage. Every time you flick off a fly, you're building more constructive thoughts. At this stage, you don't need to be convinced, just constructive and confident. Just practise uncluttering your mind of doubt and be receptive to results and lasting change.

Think of something that you've overcome and seen through to the end, even when it was tough. Right, you did that – and so you can do this

## 2. VISUALIZE LIFE, NOT JUST LOOKS

Visualizing success works. It may feel a bit 'woo-woo' to you, but I suspect in some ways you do it naturally anyway. You may not be aware of it, just honing or evoking it to reach your potential. You can practise visualizing your goals – just make sure you're not creating a dream of you standing in a Red Dress. The Red Dress is a visual, but it's a static picture of you and won't necessarily be enough to evoke a feeling, a mood which throws back an emotional response to you – encouraging you to push forward or more importantly know exactly where you are going. In the past, I've done a White Bikini visual – and it did work – but it had a distinct mood, sense, attitude to it, so crystal clear that when I reached that moment, I had the most profound sense of déjà-vu. Attach a feeling to it and you have a physical reaction which impels you forward.

In your mind, run through the course of a day, perhaps in six weeks, six months or even a year's time. Plant yourself firmly in that day. Now pin down precisely how you want to live and feel that day. I think making it a 'school day' is important and not a holiday, as it's how we spend most of our time. Focus on all the moments of the day. Waking up – how does it feel? What do you do next? Think about the order of your day and if that's too unpredictable, think about how you feel, actually embedded in your revised lifestyle. Think about all the aspects of your day and how you would love it to feel. That's the gritty stuff that really motivates us to change.

Forget what others are thinking of you. It's all about your perception, the sensations you feel – make them so compelling that whatever great feelings are stimulated, they're strong enough to recall over and over again and deter you from staying outside the circle too long. It can motivate you through the toughest of days, but if you don't know what it is you can't reach it. And your motivation is only needed for so long, until habits kick in and take over.

Of course, what you want to look like matters. It has profound influence on our mood and confidence. Vanity is the prime motivating factor for most of us – I totally get that. So thoroughly define your new aesthetic. See it and believe with unwavering confidence that the result is coming your way. Perhaps it's as simple as wearing a pair of jeans and a white t-shirt, showing your arms. Where are you? Who are you with? What are you doing? Really visualize yourself in that moment and notice what state of mind you're in. Firmly plant yourself in those clothes and feel the moment.

Perhaps you're doing an activity in clothes that you would shy away from now and you've a new confidence to lean into something that makes you feel fulfilled and full of pride. If you can pin your purpose onto something much greater and inherently meaningful, this purpose is going to propel you so powerfully beyond a weight, a dress size, a dress.

If you focus solely on a number on a scale or a dress size, you risk feeding the 'diet ghost' of your past. 'I want to be a size x' is a bit like saying 'I want to be happy'. It's too vague. Way, way too vague and it's not going to help you. A dog is happy licking its balls. I suspect you want more. I'm not saying getting into an outfit that makes your heart beat faster doesn't matter – it matters to all of us. See it, keep bringing it to mind and strive towards it but not at the expense of looking at the bigger picture.

Trust me on this; if you focus on the vision of your new lifestyle and it's one that really makes you feel fabulous about yourself, the body transformation will just happen anyway. The aesthetic is the side-effect of your new lifestyle. And you need to be able to see both of these visions in technicolour – and bring them into the forefront of your mind so often, that when you arrive there, I promise it will almost feel like you've been there before. It's worked for me and thousands of others, and I firmly believe you attract what you feel and think about most. So this week just start the practice of visualization, which is going to feel bizarre at first but then develop into absolute clarity. It could just be the oomph towards a staggering life turnaround which is permanent – and that's just what I want for you. Make it bold, beautiful and meaningful.

## 3. CONNECT THE WHYS

Given we know that there are going to be obstacles, you've got to really connect WHY BOTHER to the WHYS. Define with absolute clarity WHY you are not only starting this programme, but WHY you want to live this programme of balance forever. Anything beginning with 'I really ought to' isn't going to cut it or carry you through the days it's drizzling outside. My WHYS have changed over the years and in regaining my post-natal body after a whopping weight gain three times it was rooted in skinny jeans and not wanting to look 'mumsy'. I didn't really think about how I wanted to live at 70, whereas I now do. I know I made it harder for myself on focusing too much on the numbers.

I can summarize my main WHY as to live a long and energetic life – but I admit that's easily forgotten when the sun's out and your best friend begs you for a glass of rosé on a Thursday after work. So my WHYS are meaningful but quite medium term, as I know the medium term will lead to long-term success. I break my WHY down into having energy for the week ahead, vitality to jump out of bed tomorrow, pain control and mobility so I sleep well, balancing my hormones so I'm not snappy, and having my habits rub off on a family of three daughters. My WHYS are very much rooted in having good energy and confidence.

This week, really think about your WHYS – your deep motivation – and jot them down where you can refer to them quickly, perhaps in the notes section on your phone. It's so much more meaningful and motivating to have a reason so compelling and life changing – aiming for a size alone is just a weight-loss number, and is just doing yourself a bit of a disservice, as you'll achieve that anyway.

If you focus on the vision of your lifestyle and it's one that really makes you feel fabulous about yourself, the body transformation will just happen anyway

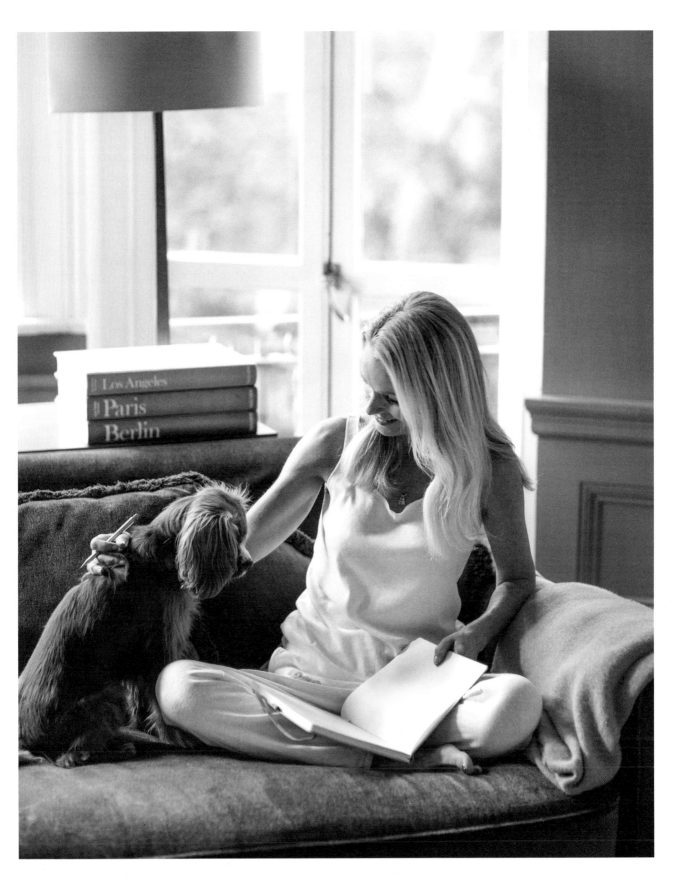

# PREPARING TO LIVE WELL

## 1. START THE DIGITAL DETOX

My tip on this one is to start straight away during your Prep Week as I am slightly fanatical about the importance of sleep. I would love you to nail this one so that you can hit the ground running with as much drive as possible in Week 1.

I'm positive that quality, regular sleep is the foundation of changing your habits and losing body fat and will pretty much support everything else you are striving for. When you sleep, your hormones are balanced and (really simply put) if they're off whack, so are you. Your appetite hormone is regulated at rest, and so if you're shattered, your will doesn't stand a chance against soaring cravings that have to do with tiredness, not lack of grub – and you're in a cranky mood. By getting ample sleep, you're getting your body to work with you on a biological level. You don't want to be relying on will alone, when your body can be working with your mind to make this phase much easier.

If you're travelling long haul, got a six-week-old baby or a snoring lover – don't give up hope. You've simply got to find a way to improve it, just really try to put habits in place to make more regular sleep happen. Whatever the circumstances. We are going to maximize your sleep, make it as regular as possible and get you to really value and enjoy it. I know the challenges and share them, but we have to find a way. Because sleep affects everything. Everything.

If you're anything like me, tiredness can totally kibosh your day, your week even. Ignore it long enough and maybe it will even wreck a month. If you're tired, you're stroppy. If you're stroppy, you're negative. If you're negative, you don't feel like aiming high but eating a chocolate croissant while moaning about how exhausted you are. After your chocolate croissant, you feel more tired. So you have a coffee. A double espresso at 4pm. You're up for a bit then crash again and can't be

bothered to workout or walk home (what's the point anyway, you've eaten a croissant – 'stinking thinking' has kicked in). So when you get home you bring the clocks forward, send the kids to bed early, order a takeaway and catch up on four episodes of something that keeps you from your bed. Then you can't sleep as you're wired from blue light and caffeine. Okay – I've embellished it a fraction but I need to hammer this point home.

The digital detox is simple and it makes so much sense – but I know it's hard to take away from what feels like 'grown-up time' that you've worked damn hard for all day. If you can get eight hours sleep per night, fantastic. It's not possible for everyone, but my absolute minimum is seven hours – which means I need eight hours in bed (because it can take me an hour to nod off, you dirty things).

You're going to refine your daily routine a bit more later on, but this week, simply set a reminder on your phone (mine has a bedtime reminder and daily alarm set for the same time each day, even at weekends) to alert you an hour before your bedtime. It usually pops up when I'm either scrolling through my phone, or on a laptop and/or watching Netflix. All this light stimulates us to stay awake and so the moment the reminder pops up – it's devices off, TV off and I go straight into my bedtime routine. My alarm is automatically set for the morning and my phone is put onto airplane mode, charged and in a drawer out of sight (a fireman told me to do this in case of an emergency, or it would be out of the room). But airplane mode is fabulous at making you feel like an idiot should you feel the need to check the news at 3am if you get up for a wee. So use it.

## 2. BRING ON THE BRAIN-NAP

Our days are so overstimulated in the modern world, no doubt about it. We're reachable 24/7 and it's a constant juggle with the demands of careers, children, home life, looking after family, let alone having time out with friends and taking pleasure in what you love.

So, before you start, I'd love you to try to brain-nap, every single day. Twenty minutes if you can – but start with ten if you're super-important. If you notice it's impossible to switch off for even ten minutes, then you really need to look at your routine. We all need a little time out each day.

Bombarded by news, emails, texts, calls and social media, we're just slammed with stimulation all day long, often not even realizing that we're fatigued by information and Things to Do. We're living in a time where we're really a social experiment and I'm seeing more and more people coming to us with anxiety or on the verge of burnout. So along with the digital detox in the evening, I'd love you to practise the brain-nap, starting today. Hell, if you can manage it, take two.

We know that meditation increases productivity and dramatically reduces stress – and if you can meditate, fabulous. If you're annoyed you still didn't get it on the third try like me, keep it this simple: lie down for whatever time you can spare and just rest (I set a soothing reminder on my phone to go off at the end of the nap – oh, the irony). That's all – clear your mind and just breathe. You'll get better at letting go of worry the more you do it. Many days it's a bit impractical for me to lie on the office floor or pavement and I suspect it'll be the same for you. So perhaps your brain-nap might be as simple as gazing out of the window of the train and not looking at your phone – allowing yourself some time just to be present, mindful and not 'wired' to screens and life on super-high speed.

It's about looking out – not down. Chin up too – it'll even help your posture. Maybe it'll be half an hour in the garden, or your daily walk could be your meditation, perhaps you're able to take ten minutes to drink your tea in the morning undisturbed. The main purpose is to UNPLUG. If we don't choose to disconnect in little nuggets throughout the day, we're opting in to information overload. The world won't stop if you take 20 minutes out for yourself. Give guilt the boot. Taking charge to destress is one step towards reducing your stress and balancing cortisol levels – so it has a physical and biological effect on your mood and health. Find your version of what works for you. Slowing down is going to speed up your results.

If we don't choose to disconnect in little nuggets throughout the day, we're opting in to information overload

# 3. CREATE A BATH & BEDTIME SANCTUARY

You have an hour between your digital detox and bedtime to unwind so make this precious hour count. It's about pampering yourself as much as you can and truly switching off from the day. Your bathroom and bedroom need to feel like your own little sanctuary – even if you're sharing it with rubber ducks.

As we switch from day to night, it's essential to be ruthless about devices. Make sure your phone is charged, airplane mode on, alarm set and it's out of sight in a drawer. Absolutely no tablets, TV or laptops – we're focusing on restoring your bedroom to a place of rest.

Take time out this week (even if it's just a ten-minute edit of both bathroom and bedroom) to clear all surfaces and surround yourself with belongings that are either practical or beautiful. Declutter as much as you can and have everything in its place. Blitz what you don't either love or need.

Clear all the surfaces of your bathroom and store all your products away or arrange them neatly on trays or in baskets. Indulge yourself with products that you know lift your mood instantly – and try to choose products that have a physical benefit and don't just look the part. I use Epsom salts which are rich in magnesium (helping muscles to relax and promoting a good night's kip). I find they really help me nod off and I usually pimp them up with some relaxing essential oils. Make a note of little luxuries that you can add to your rewards list for later in your reset.

Keep your bedroom as a place of restoration and sleep. Tidy your bedside drawers and banish all electrical devices from your room. Make sure you clear away piles of clutter reminding you of things to do. Once you've restored your bedroom and bathroom, don't allow chaos to build up. You can do this bit by bit – but the sooner you take delight in this hour of your day, the sooner you'll come to really look forward to it and give up the remote.

Pop a couple of blooms in a little glass by your bed. A little tray to keep rings, hand cream, a pillow mist and lip balm is all you need. Invest in lovely linens and beautiful books with proper paper pages. Keep the temperature low and make sure you have blackout curtains and no little lights glowing to get the deepest sleep.

I hope you feel your shoulders drop once you switch into bedtime hour and wake up in what should feel like a sanctuary. Take a mental snapshot in your mind each night to just give yourself that reminder to spruce things up when the clutter builds and beauty fades a little. It's one precious hour, so up the bliss factor to help you mentally and physically unplug from the world and prepare you for a restful, deep sleep. Your surroundings have such a profound impact on your mood and ability to unplug from the day and can help you enjoy much more sleep.

I promise that in a couple of weeks, you will be feeling dramatically better. It's about getting back to old-fashioned habits. Sound sleep is the absolute foundation on which you are going to build the rest of your habits. We all deserve an hour for ourselves in the evening and spending that slowing down from the pace that we all live at is so valuable – you'll soon feel the benefit of that hour well spent.

# Keep your bedroom a place of restoration and sleep

# PREPARING TO EAT BEAUTIFULLY

## 1. SWOT UP ON THE PRINCIPLES

To really buy into anything, yet alone invest time and effort in it, you have to get it and believe it. Spend as much time as you can this week in understanding the principles of Eating Beautifully. Once you grasp the simple science and logic behind the importance of eating whole food, little and often – and balancing out the protein, low-GI carbs and good fats – you are far more likely to start strong and stick at it. Knowing the effect that hidden sugars will have on your mood and appetite, for example, will really help you get the importance of giving up the granola bar in the morning. If you realize that it's going to spike your blood-sugar levels, cause a mid-morning slump and appetite surge, you're more likely to invest a few minutes in the evening planning a speedy and healthy breakfast which can have a positive impact on your whole day.

There's heaps more information and background for you in my first book, *The Louise Parker Method: Lean for Life* for further reading. Spend some time reading about the effect of sugar on just about every aspect of your health and look into how good fats and sufficient protein help you maintain good health and a healthy weight. Education is power – and so swot up if you have time, or just take my word for it – and see how dramatically different you feel in a few weeks.

These are the basic principles of our Food Plan:

- It's neither low carb, high protein or super-high in fat – it's simply a balance of food groups from the most nutritious sources possible, keeping it real and do-able.

- You'll aim to eat three meals and two snacks per day. This balances your macronutrients (that's protein, low-GI carbohydrates and good fats) throughout the day. It spreads your calorific intake so that you maintain good blood-sugar balance, which turns that 'fat-burning tap' on and manages your hormones. We all know that good hormonal balance keeps mood good, appetite in calm control and your concentration at its best.

- Each meal will have a delicate amount of protein, low-GI carbs (sometimes sturdier ones like wholemeal bread, porridge and high-fibre crackers) but primarily heaps of vegetables and a good balance of the lower-sugar fruit. By eliminating refined carbs and even many of the medium-GI carbs in the Transform Phase, you take on board heaps of low-GI carbs – which means that volume wise, you have more fibre, water, vitamins and minerals. We're not cutting out the carbs – we're just selecting the carbs that are packed full of nutrients and don't give you a blood-sugar high. It means that each day we are packing in as much fibre and vitamins that we can. Later in the Balance Phase, we reintroduce more grains – but for now we want you getting creative with heaps more veggies. It's a great habit to get into and resets your appetite and style of eating.

- Portions matter – and most of the work is done for you here in the recipes. Stick to them as closely as you can, but there's no need to be obsessive about it. Do bear in mind that the portions in the recipes are based on the nutritional needs of the average woman, and are not personally adjusted to you as one of our dieticians would if you were following a supported programme. Trust your appetite and listen to your gut (no pun intended) because if you're a triathlete, you're going to need way more fuel than someone who's perhaps light on muscle and new to exercise. More veg than is in a recipe isn't going to affect your results, so add some more if you like. Don't be afraid to interchange and experiment with them either to suit your taste – just remember to avoid the sugars and the obvious no-nos. I love to see you changing things up and experimenting, as it engages you and you're more likely to get into lasting change.

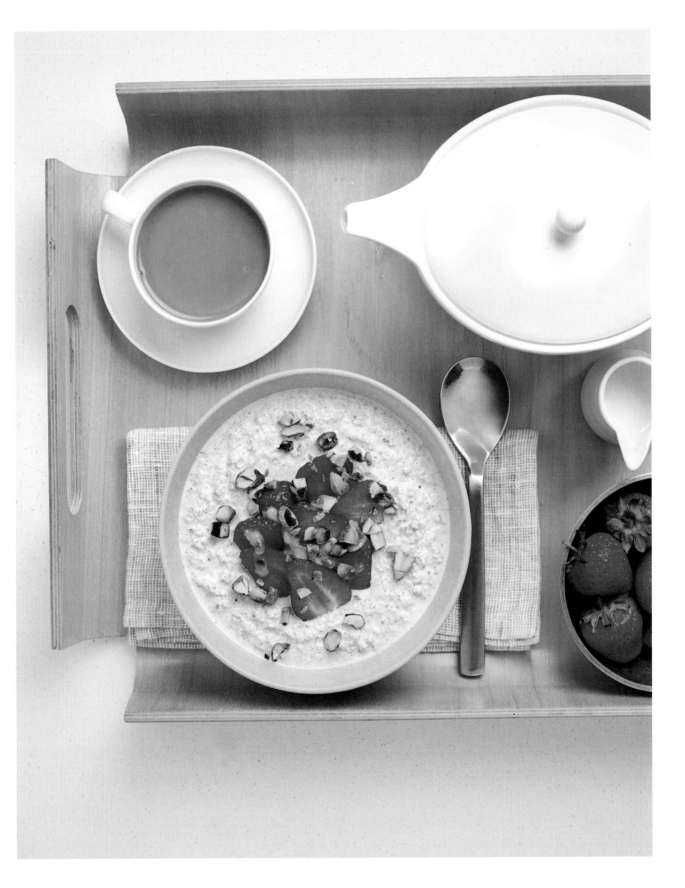

## 2. SCRAP THE SUGAR

Sugar – refined, hidden or organic – is the enemy of your success on the plan. We all know why – and so I'm suggesting you start to Scrap the Sugar in your Prep Week. It actually makes for a much gentler, kinder kick-off, where your mood will already be on the up and appetite much more in sync. You won't be doing yourself any favours if you say a long goodbye to Ben and Jerry this week – just call it quits as soon as you can. It's a big task for most and so just do the best you can. You needn't be squeaky clean, but the more distance between you and your last sugar hit, the easier the ride, I promise.

Don't worry too much about the timing of your meals or too many of the other details – just simply scrap the sugar as much as you can. So we're talking all the obvious cakes, biscuits, 'healthy' granola bars, cereals and (sorry) booze. You'll find that by eliminating sugar, you're just naturally going to pick up whole foods to eat and you're going to up your hydration too as you put down the wine. Please don't fret if you don't do it absolutely – I'm just really advising you to reduce it as much as you can, to make next week simpler for you. I also want you to notice how you quite quickly feel very well again, in just a matter of days.

By suggesting you give up sugar in the Prep Week, I'm shrewdly stopping you self-sabotaging and having a 'last hurrah', whacking on 2kg of weight before Week 1 and mentally reinforcing that you are 'starting a diet' – which you are not. Don't forget that you're not giving up sugar or booze forever. This phase is a temporary period in which you give them the boot as best you can to give your new habits the best chance to form as your tastes change too. The very reason we cut out the sugar for a decent period

of time is firstly, to get the result you want, but essentially so that you lose the taste for it and learn a new way. And then, when you're thrilled with the results, the foods that are worth their sugar will come back in the Balance Phase – but more about this later. So just ease into it this week – no need to eat all the croissants as if the country is running out of them. Although with Brexit, I may have a point.

Long term, I'm not recommending that you live in a home that has nothing but whole, organic food in it. A few weeks from now, I hope that you can keep beautiful biscuits for guests in the house, without them winking at you. We've got to be able to live around foods that are not strictly on Method, as it's just part and parcel of normal life, where sweets are piled high at every checkout. So, you've got to get used to having sugar around you as it's everywhere. However, if you are someone who struggles with sugar addiction, then I do suggest you make it easier for yourself and give the cupboards at home a good clear out. It's a good exercise too in seeing where hidden sugars lurk. Spend an hour going through the fridge and store cupboard and check the labels for hidden sugars. I'd need a double-page spread to list the surprising culprits, so read the labels and just ditch the things you know will tempt you most when you're bored or stressed. Start with what you know to be your weakest link – for example, I know I can't keep sugared almonds at home. I don't live in a sugar-free house, however, but this comes later once you've kicked the habit.

I think that's a big enough task for this week. Please don't leave just yet…

# 3. SIMPLE PLANNING & STOCK UP

Over the three books I've written (and you can use any of the recipes in all my books for your Transform Phase – interchanging all the main meals for either lunch or supper) you'll find a total of 58 breakfasts, 60 snacks and 140 main meals. There really is a colossal choice, but I don't want to overwhelm you with all of them straight off.

As the weeks tick by, I'll be nudging you to keep changing up your repertoire and love your new style of eating – to keep you interested, inventive and not narrowing down what you eat too much. More on this later.

This week, have a good flick through the recipes and just mark the ones that jump out at you, perhaps choosing some of the faster recipes and ones that are easy to batch-cook – saving you time in the next week. In time you're going to ring the changes but just bear in mind that our prime goal is to get you settled into a style of eating that you actually really love. So choose meals you just know you'll enjoy – you've got to find the joy in it from Week 1.

Just don't overcomplicate it and choose too many to shop for and prepare as you'll feel consumed by it and there's plenty else to be getting on with. My tip is to choose no more than two or three breakfasts, four quick snacks and about six main meals that you can either batch-cook or use leftovers. That's all. You'll be cooking up a storm otherwise. Keep the food preparation as simple as you can this week. Once you're settled in, you can look into hundreds of other recipes I have for you.

So – simply find a handful of meals that really appeal to you and stock up on the ingredients so that you're good to go.

Next week, you're going to get into regular meal planning which I admit sounds dull, but makes your life so much more relaxed. It becomes quite effortless once you're living this way – it just needs some planning in the early weeks. You also waste far less food. I don't do formal weekly menu planning, but I stock up the fridge with foods that are on Method and from there I know we can concoct an array of meals each week, even if time is tight.

I also suggest preparing for those days that you are unprepared and caught short of ingredients. There will be days you've forgotten to shop, are home late, even your hair is tired and the only items in your fridge are a head of broccoli, some milk and a few eggs. So when you do your first big shop, make sure you buy ingredients that have a good fridge life so that you're easily able to throw together fit, fast food on days that the flesh feels a bit unwilling. Grab, too, a handful of things that you can keep in the pantry and freezer – so you always have something to throw together that's fast and full of flavour. There is absolutely nothing wrong with eating the right kinds of frozen or tinned foods. Here are my top items (not including condiments, spices and so on) that I keep stocked because I know I can concoct a good handful of meals from them within minutes:

- Fridge: eggs, firm tofu, feta cheese, Parmesan, mature Cheddar, olives, cured ham, lactose-free milk (it lasts), yogurt

- Freezer: mixed berries, raspberries, cherries, peas, mixed veg, ready-chopped onions, fresh herbs, spinach, edamame beans

- Store cupboard: canned lentils, canned beans (kidney, cannellini and butter beans), canned chickpeas, canned tuna in oil, canned tomatoes, dried lentils, cannellini beans, chickpeas, oatbran, nut butters

# PREPARING TO WORK OUT INTELLIGENTLY

## 1. SCHEDULE IN YOUR DAILY RENT

Part of your Prep Week is reading through the book from start to finish, so you won't be surprised by anything as you enter into a new week. Everything I have set out for you in terms of workouts is the ideal – but please don't not start or toss it aside if you think you can only achieve half of it. This is perfectionism preventing you from succeeding – so just aim to do as much as you can.

You can only do what you can do – just try. You'll find that your motivation gathers pace as you go. We are trying to build the space, routine and habit of exercise – and of course it's going to be an adjustment. Just aim for your personal best for now – you have a lifetime to build and adjust your routine. So, even if your rent is tiny one day – you're tired and it's drizzling outside – by simply going for a walk or doing a few mobility stretches you will remind yourself that you are someone who is active. We're training your brain as much as your body and, after a while, it will feel just natural to move daily. This is why I always refer to 'daily rent' as it prevents the start/stop mentality – it just keeps the habit alive.

The biggest barrier is TIME (and basically not wanting to do it, or start it) so we are going to nail this right now, if what you want is long-term habit change. We have to reclaim your workout times before we start. Overcome this today and you're already getting into a can-do mindset. See the obstacles and find a way. I'm assuming you want to become someone who exercises regularly, not obsessively, and that you want it to become a really strong part of your New Normal.

It's easy to say we have no time to exercise, but we have to find a way through this hurdle. It's not easy to carve out the time, especially if you're a single mum, working two jobs, looking after ageing parents. I get it. But – if you are the lifeline to so many people, even more reason to help yourself first. Remember, making yourself a priority is not indulgent, it's necessary. I'm not preaching to you, rather giving myself a reminder too. If we ignore ourselves, we are literally saying we are not worth it, so let's find the time, because we are. I know it's not easy, but I never promised that getting started was easy. What I am promising is that once you have the habit and the unfamiliar becomes familiar, it really does get easier. Or 80 per cent easier – and I'm sure you'd settle for that.

Your challenge this first six weeks is, whatever else is going on around you, to find the time to train. Facts like 'a 30-minute workout is just over 2 per cent of your day' are damn irritating because you can't argue with it – it's fact. You have to work out if your goal of being someone strong and healthy is worth 2 per cent of your day. You know it is – we've just got to get you into it. If you can't find the time, you're saying you're not a priority. Throughout this Prep Week, just be conscious of where you are wasting time. What can you take out of your day to make the space?

I've devised the workouts to be as time effective as possible and the idea of being more active all of the time – weaving those steps in – hopefully means that you notice it less than you would if you were driving to a gym to walk on a treadmill for an hour. Yawn.

You need to schedule in the following per week for the first two weeks:

- Four sessions of 40 minutes to work out at home (to allow time to grasp the moves and stretch)

- Times throughout the week you can weave your walking in, and a good long walk at the weekend to catch up on your step count, if you need to (ideally making it social and bringing along family and friends)

That's all you need to do for now. At the end of each fortnight, as you move into another phase, you're going to schedule in the next two weeks too.

What I am promising
is that once you
have the habit and
the unfamiliar
becomes familiar,
it really does
get easier

## 2. CREATE YOUR SPACE

You can save so much time with at-home workouts (rather than travelling to a gym), but it takes discipline and you do need to 'nest' a space before you start. If I'm not training in my studio, or in the park, I'm doing a 20–40-minute routine at home. Some days it may just be six minutes stretching – just something to keep me in the habit. I don't have a spare room, but I have a regular space that I go to – and I take two minutes, if that, to set it up. I keep a box in my sitting room with various toys and gadgets – which you can add into your routine later. Your environment affects your mood and motivation hugely, so don't expect this habit to feel good unless you put some care into it. Lie on a grubby kitchen floor with the dog licking your face, and you're setting yourself up to fail.

I shut the door, make it clear to everyone at home it's my time, sort out a play list (I have a dozen ready prepped of different lengths), roll out my yoga mat and light a citrus-scented candle – just this small effort marks it as my time and just makes it feel like a treat and not a chore. If you can, have a full-length mirror handy (and I've planned my space around this) as it really helps with checking your form.

On days it's warm, I go outside – but find your own little training territory. There's something about the routine and familiarity of it that helps keep you in the habit of returning to your little 'workout space'. I've been doing it so long now that I've learned to keep going through pony-tail and homework dilemmas. When my scented candle runs out, I feel pleased that I've burned through so many workouts and treat myself to another. So this week, create your space and make it quick to set up each time.

## 3. GET KITTED OUT

This is partly practical and partly about putting a swagger in your step. You will probably want to treat yourself to a whole new wardrobe once you're six or twelve weeks in, but before we start your reset, take an hour to clear out your cupboards and make sure that you've got the basics for exercising. Anything badly fitting that makes your heart sink a bit, give to charity. You need very little kit to begin exercising so no need to spend a fortune, but I think it's important you wear clothing that is fitted and makes you feel good. I know it's hard when you perhaps feel insecure about your body and are used to hiding under baggy clothes. I find that compression leggings allow you to connect to your body – you're somehow able to feel the muscles contract more than if you're slobbing about in baggy layers that have seen better days. It's also just good to see the shape of your body and accept what needs work – it will help you visually track your progress and spur you on.

You're going to be training inside and outside so you need to be set up for both. You need a couple of pairs of good leggings, two decent sports bras, a couple of tank tops and long-sleeved tops for walking outside, sports socks, a decent pair of cross trainers and something to throw over you when you need a waterproof. That's it. High street stores do brilliant affordable options now, but if you're going to invest in just three items, make it good compression leggings, a good bra and trainers (and seek advice on these). The rest you can skimp on.

Give some thought to what you're going to be wearing when you're doing the extra walking too – you may need new trainers and to adjust your clothing for this. If I'm not prepped in this department it's my best excuse to get a taxi home rather than walk – so plan what you need to get those extra steps in.

## 4. MEASURE YOUR MOVEMENT

Living the Method isn't about just doing workouts – it's about weaving as much movement into your life as possible. So, it's about walking more, gardening, spending more active time with your family and basically getting your steps in. Your body is designed to move; we're just not designed to sit for as long as we do. I've seen 70-year-old bodies who've always gardened or walked or ridden horses that are more powerful than young gym bunnies who drive to a treadmill – your lifestyle of activity is going to profoundly change your body in time.

You may have to get yourself out of a rut and it's as much about willingness, honing that discipline, preparing and practising until the desire to move does take over (with the odd shove). If activity and walking just don't come easily to you the only way round it is to just get on with it until the unfamiliar feels familiar.

For your Prep Week I want you to begin measuring your weekly movement with a tracker (not your phone, as it isn't always on you). Using a movement tracker is really useful in the short term – most of us tend to think we move more than we do. I do think you can get a bit obsessed with them and my steal on this is to borrow one for the next few weeks – just so you know that you're

stepping in the right direction. I wore one for a month a couple of years ago and now have a clear idea of what I need to do to achieve my 100,000 steps per week. It's not actually easy, especially in winter. Every now and then, I'll whack the tracker back on again for a week when I need a motivational boost. You'll be surprised how many steps you do at home and running about the office – they don't all need to be on dedicated walks. It's really helpful in the short term and surprising to see how much you can weave in just doing housework at home at the weekend – not that this motivates me much.

We're going to ease your steps up from a minimum of 45,000 a week to 70,000 but don't throw the towel in if you don't reach the target each week – it's really there to remind you to simply move more and get a new routine going. If your weekly count is still low by Friday, you can make up some progress at the weekend (but please don't go out walking for hours). So, either borrow or buy a tracker this week and make sure it's set up and good to go. As the weeks go on, I'm going to set you challenges to get your daily steps up. We're going to monitor it for the first six weeks, until it becomes a habit.

Living the Method isn't just about doing workouts – it's about weaving as much movement into your life as possible

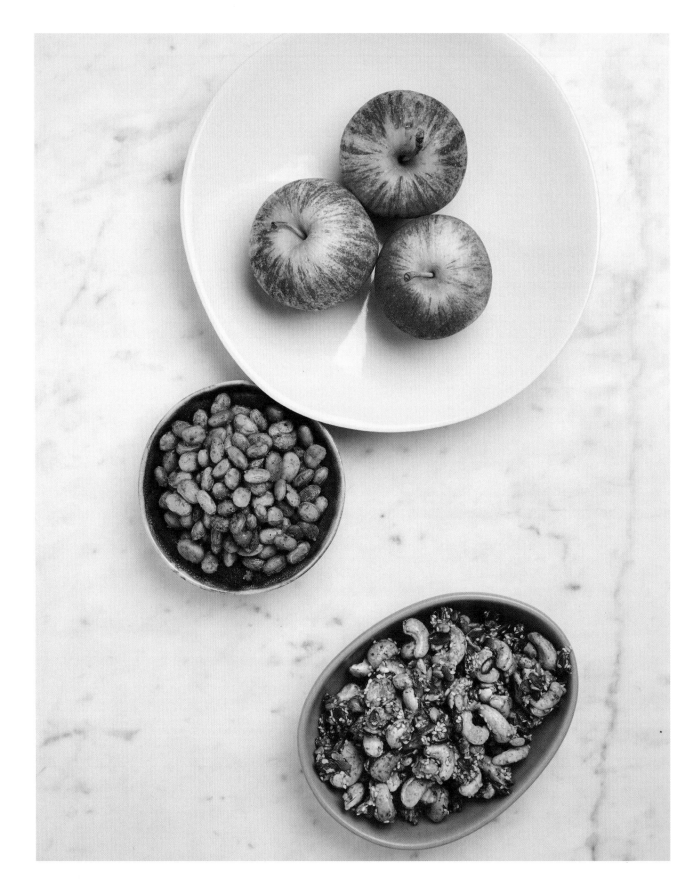

# PREP WEEK CHECKLIST

☐ Keep an open mind. Practise decluttering your mind from self-doubt.

☐ Start the practice of visualization – try the visualisation of a day sometime in the future and define your new aesthetic activity.

☐ Really think about your *whys* – your deep motivations. Jot them down where you can refer to them quickly.

☐ Start the digital detox. Set a reminder to put away your phone an hour before bed. Use airplane mode.

☐ Try to brain-nap for 20 minutes every single day – however works for you.

☐ Use the hour before bed to create a bath and bedtime sanctuary – declutter the space of electrical devices and replace them with things you love.

☐ Swot up on the principles of Eating Beautifully. You can refer to my first book *The Louise Parker Method: Lean for Life* for more information. Start to Scrap the Sugar – begin with your weakest link and begin to clear your cupboards of items with hidden sugar.

☐ Flick through any of my books and mark a handful of meals that really appeal to you.

☐ Stock up your store cupboard, fridge and freezer with key ingredients for when you're unprepared on busier days.

☐ Schedule in your workout times – four sessions of 40 minutes to work out at home and times throughout the week when you can weave in your walking.

☐ Create your workout space at home – make it quick to set up each time.

☐ Begin measuring your movement with a tracker (not your phone because it's not on you all the time).

WEEK

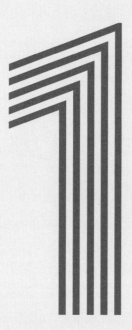

I'm so excited for you and I hope you're raring to go. Start with utter conviction that you can devote yourself to this programme, regardless of what your track record is. You're going to reset habits for a happier, healthier life and you're going to get staggering results with it. And they're going to go far beyond the aesthetic. You're going to claim back your energy and overhaul your lifestyle – you'll never want to go back.

I know that anyone can have success with the programme, because I've witnessed it thousands of times. But you do have to throw yourself in fully. What I know for sure is the more you engage in all the pillars, the easier the whole programme clicks together and becomes a pleasure to follow. The more you do, the easier it gets. Don't half-arse it. Dedicate these weeks to making life changes that last.

Believe you can and you are half way there. That's not to say you have to do everything 'perfectly' – but catch yourself when you wander off track and learn to jump back into the middle of the circle. And the longer you spend in the middle of the circle, the hardier your habits will be – and the stronger the habit, the more impressive the result. And the real joy is that it's truly sustainable.

Whatever your reason for starting the Method, I'm thrilled you're about to begin and I hope that it changes your life as it has mine. Here's to being fit, happy and free.

# THINK SUCCESSFULLY

## BE ACCOUNTABLE, TO YOU & YOUR TRIBE

It helps immensely to be accountable – primarily to yourself, but also to someone you know will support you, or even a tribe of people who share your intentions. You'll find it a real rod for your motivation in the early days. I know it's a ginormous part of the equation of the success of our programmes. Our dieticians at Louise Parker are degree qualified and have specialist training – but above all they're skilled at motivating, inducing behavioural change and good old-fashioned accountability. Your dietician coaches you beyond the finish line and into the Lifestyle Phase, with exceptional knowledge, and helps you tweak and challenge your behaviours and thought, kindly and through every obstacle – whether that be medical, lifestyle or headspace. It's about motivating you through the tougher weeks and keeping you consistent.

Ultimately, it's about being answerable to yourself, propelling you forward, always moving forward – even if it's just an inch. I used the term 'Tribal Transformation' when I was writing my first book. I nearly deleted it as I found it a bit naff, but I'm so glad I didn't. I meant for readers to go and find their Tribe, thinking they'd grab a couple of mates and a sister or neighbour, book-club style, to help motivate them through the Transform Phase.

Over the last three years, a phenomenal – and I mean phenomenal – group of followers has gathered on social media (Instagram in particular) under #leanietribe #louiseparkermethod. They have formed friendships and solidarity and it's given me sweaty eyeballs. They are the absolute definition of a Tribe. They meet up, they share a purpose, fears, blips and victories – united by their shared goal. I urge you to find your Tribe or join ours and we will encourage you. And then when it's 'clicked' for you, maybe you could pass it on.

You may bore your best friends if you message them daily to say you're about to work out, you've completed your workout, you've prepped your snacks or got 7½ hours sleep with only one wee wake-up. I know this would irritate me more than those 'Mandy has lost her sock, please stop your busy life and look for my child's sock in your child's rucksack' emails that bring up words that are not suitable for print.

But if you find a little group of people who are trying to make changes just like you, lean on them, tell them what you're aiming for this week, what you may be finding difficult and need help with – and be totally honest – you'll be amazed by how your sharing will be reciprocated back and forth like a little game of inspirational ping pong. Give it away, and you'll receive it back.

Align yourself with those who share your positivity as you want to lift up those who are really trying for themselves – do not waste your energy on someone who is persistently moaning and 'stinking thinking'. We're all allowed some down days on the Pity Pot, but too much time there and you're going to end up stuck there. Keep careful company and surround yourself with those who have your back and do the same for them.

I suggest you pick a time each week – Sunday evenings might work well – to just take stock for 15 minutes. Your accountability check needn't turn into a massive time drain. Simply stop and reflect on the week that's gone. You don't need to have all the answers this week – but by being persistent with a weekly accountability check, I'm damn sure you're going to succeed. If you're not aware of what you're doing, you simply can't change it.

What do you need to adjust for next week to improve your habits with ease? What have you had difficulty with and how can you simply shift it around? Is there something you are slacking off? Work out why and fix it fast. Nip it in the bud. Recognize the obstacles that you're going to have to look at. I hope you find a Tribe, that they spur you on and that you regularly check in with them and yourself, as you would a friend. Be honest, constructive and kind.

## KEEP IT IN THE DAY

Six weeks can seem like an age in Week 1, but it's going to go as quick as a tick. Think back to what you were doing this time six weeks ago. Scary, isn't it? For this little chapter – or two or three – of your life, you're going to need to summon some motivation and that I know can be daunting. I just want to reassure you that you're not going to have to hold on with sheer grit for 42 days. You can do this – and it's heaps easier than you think. The idea is that you won't have to grasp on to motivation and summon it up ten times a day forever. Nope. As the days tick by, you'll need less and less of it to fuel you, you'll just start running on autopilot.

I've bombarded you with words like 'forever', 'longevity' and overused the word 'habit' already, I know, I know, I know. I like repetition because it works. Chances are you're starting out this week with a reasonable level of apprehension and perhaps you're doubtful about whether this will work for you. Maybe motivation is feeling a bit shaky as you've yet to prove to yourself that you can see a plan through from start to finish. (The trick here, is that it never really finishes…)

I strongly believe that motivation is a temporary wave to propel you towards your goal until routines take over and become an instinctive part of you. We simply can't rely on motivation forever – imagine how exhausted you'd be? I intend to get you to your New Normal where you just become this more active person, someone who eats better and looks after themself – for the majority of the time. Because you like it and it works and it just feels normal and good. Like feeding your dog. Or not stealing from sweet shops. You don't have to motivate yourself to do that, you just do it. You won't be a health bore and you're not going to be obsessed about your lifestyle. You'll find the balance. You'll still party and eat cake and sip rosé on hot summer days.

In the back of your mind, make sure you're not projecting scepticism from some fad you did last summer, which left you tired, irritable, hungry and quitting. The Method is different and if you keep practising it, just the best you possibly can – one day at a time, then a week and give it time – it just clicks into place. Motivation and steely determination won't need to prop you up. Lifestyle becomes natural. Genuinely, just inherent.

And if it's truly difficult for you to sustain it or you're not practising part of the Method, that can be fixed (it's usually a case of an 'on and off again' mindset, or not really taking on board the habits).

So rest assured, keep an open mind that this 'click' will take place. I've literally just received a message from a client to say it's just 'clicked' (couldn't make it up if I tried – hello Jo) and she is ecstatic, one year on. I know there's effort and planning and graft to put in over the coming weeks (and I've done it myself so I truly get it) so my tip this week is so basic. Keep it in the day. I know this sounds at odds with planning ahead and visualizing, but once that's done, just aim to keep the motivation going one day at a time. Don't project ahead about your doubt in motivation or worry how tricky it might be tomorrow. It may just be way easier than you think.

So your main goal, each day, is just to get your head on the pillow each night (at a decent hour) and tick off the day. Don't count them too obsessively – wear the days lightly so you can feel yourself just easing into a new way of doing things. And don't overcomplicate it. You're just trying to be more positive, eat more wisely, live a bit better and move. Keep it simple and in the day and know that you won't have to rely on motivation forever.

# LIVE WELL

## ROUTINE RECCE

In the Prep Week you've hopefully started your digital detox, bed and bathtime routine, and scheduled in your workouts. So already you're shining a light on your diary and being aware of where you spend your time. Given this is your lifestyle overhaul, it makes sense to start by looking at how things stand today, so that as the weeks progress, you can mould your lifestyle into one that works for you on many levels.

It's bizarre, really, to think how much we do each week, yet we propel ourselves from one activity to the next – and never really stop to see where we are spending our most valuable commodity. Easy to say and oh so easy to overlook. We know where we spend our cash – the drains, the investments – but we rarely stop and really look at where our time goes. And we need to reclaim some time, redistribute it and invest this commodity wisely.

I take stock of my diary every six weeks, coinciding with school terms, so it feels more manageable. I look at the weeks ahead and the first thing I do is put in all the non-negotiables. I put everything in – work, travel time, waking time, breakfast time, eight minutes' make-up time, the lot. I try to batch and create patterns and routines wherever they emerge as I know if I have a floating 'ought to do that' in my diary, it's going to get eaten by an urgent something. There is always something. Diarize it and stick to it. Workouts go in daily, same time during the week and the same time at

weekends – I know I'll have to drop two or three, so I end up with four – that's fine. I batch time for emails so I don't waste time checking them 50 times a day. Batch, batch, batch and create a routine to save you so much time.

Only if you review it can you change it and tweak it to a routine that works for you and your family. Remember that we're creating a habit shift so we want as much routine as possible. And I can assure you that life won't be boring – it throws ample surprises and opportunities – but we just want to compose your weeks as close to how you'd like them to roll as possible.

Assuming you're busy during the day with either parenting or work or both, you have weekday morning and evening routines which are, to a certain extent, under your control. And weekends that are probably more flexible. There are responsibilities you'll have that you can't move – like turning up at work and picking children up from school.

In half-hour sections, have a look at your morning routine, from the time you wake up to the time your first commitment starts. Do the same with your evening routine – from the time you get home to the time you turn your lights out.

You don't have to totally redesign your lifestyle this week, just know where you're spending your life. More tweaks come later as you ease into the programme.

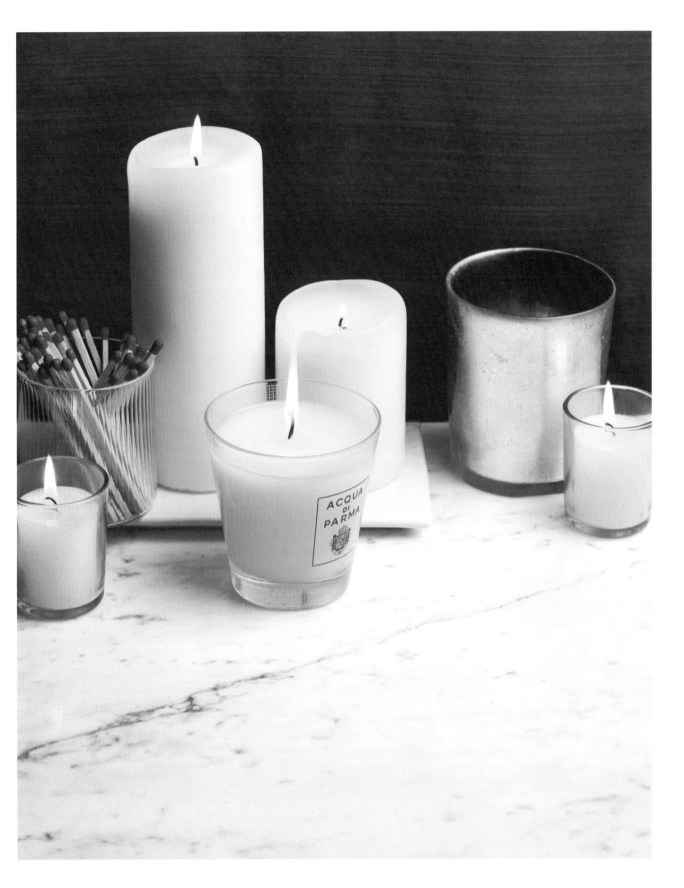

## HERE ARE SOME TIPS:

- Divide your morning and evening routine into half-hour sections and examine them.

- Look at your routine – day by day, hour by hour – and just be aware of where you're spending your time.

- Make sure you have the three routines mentioned on the previous page popped in – digital detox, bedtime and your workout time.

- Highlight what you don't like and what you have the ability to change.

- Just start thinking about what shifts you can make as you go about your week.

- What are the biggest drains on your time (that don't serve you or your family)?

- Think about what jobs you can batch to save more time.

- Where can you ask for help and redistribute the load? You cannot do it all.

## YOU MIGHT WANT TO CARVE OUT TIME FOR:

- A good breakfast at the table to start the day off well, unrushed.

- Some simple food preparation for the day or evening.

- Getting your movement in, ideally combining it with other jobs.

- Time to relax and destress.

- Time to do nothing – just free time. Every schedule needs wiggle room.

Keep this in the front of your mind and written down, so that you can keep adding to it. Once you've completed the first fortnight, it will be a practical help to take further stock and drive a routine that's balanced, healthy and most of all sustainable. Ultimately you want to find pleasure in the ebb and flow of your week. Align the lifestyle habits with pleasure and they'll be sticky.

We are going to refine this in Week 6 once your programme is underway – but this week, I simply want you to start thinking about the best possible routine you can make for yourself.

## STRESS-TESTING YOUR LANGUAGE

We are going to get a handle on diminishing stress as much as possible. It's a tall order, I know. Life seems to be getting busier and faster and more demanding for all of us, whatever our age, career or lifestyle.

But you've already set some good foundations in your Prep Week which, given a bit of time and consistency, are going to work wonders. It's important to pay attention to when stress pops up, peak times and how you can get a handle on it.

But what we do know – and notice all the time with hundreds of clients – is that when we get sleep, rest and stress in much better sync, all the other habits genuinely click into place so much easier. The positive effect of manipulating our hormones to work with us and not against us is phenomenal. So calming life down – through some simple changes – is going to get you the optimal results in the swiftest way possible.

The good news is, if we get a real handle on resting, reviving and seriously paying attention to lessening the stress in our lives, our hormonal health improves and can do so at a really impressive rate.

Our dieticians coach so much more than what to and what not to eat. By mentoring each client to make practical, sustainable lifestyle changes, the key factors of eating well and training consistently become enjoyable and last. Think back to the four-legged stool – each pillar supports the other, so Eat Beautifully and Work Out Intelligently aren't going to come easily or remain sticky if you ignore Live Well.

To put it simply, you're already starting to manage your cortisol levels (the stress hormone) by easing off devices, chilling out more and getting regular sleep. You're also balancing your levels of the hormone ghrelin (which manages your appetite) through more regular sleep. So already those two are helping you, without having to white knuckle it on discipline alone. Increasing your rest time is going to help prevent adrenal fatigue, too. And because you're calmer and sleeping well, you're in a much chirpier mood, making you more likely to slip on your trainers and go to release some endorphins (happy hormones) through exercise. This in turn causes stress to plummet further so you're much more likely to eat well and keep insulin (the hormone that balances your blood-sugar levels) under control.

You're going to tackle the bigger stresses in Week 3. This week, your priority is your digital detox, bedtime routine and brain-naps. You can obsess over those a bit because they're absolutely key.

I also want you to try this – and it's not as easy as it sounds. Pay close attention to the language you use – in conversation with yourself and others. Simply delete the word 'stress' from your vocabulary. When you run around saying 'I'm so stressed', you're reinforcing that feeling – you're revving it up, amplifying it and reminding your brain to panic and release more adrenalin and cortisol (depleting you further). And equally as important, risk boring people with competitive stress syndrome.

I'm not saying tape your jaw, but just rephrase your language to something that's going to motivate and not deplete you. 'It's a challenge, but I'm on it'. That sort of thing. Put a coin in a jar every time you complain – save it for your Rewards Week.

# EAT BEAUTIFULLY

## MEAL PLANNING

Meal planning will become instinctive and I don't want you tied to menus like a 1950s housewife but, and especially if you're super-busy, you'll gain back time spent on choosing a good outline of the week's menu and shopping ahead.

Do more if you can, but really don't stress if you're experimenting at a slower pace – you have years to try all of the recipes. In Week 4, I'm going to take you out of your comfort zone and ask you to change it all up.

Having got the basic ingredients in for this week and stocked up for emergencies in Prep Week, it's time to introduce planning time once a week. Just for the first six weeks, set aside 30 minutes to choose what you're going to introduce and list what you need. Your mood is going to dictate what you feel like eating any given day, which is why I think it's crucial to have some basics stocked for when you don't feel like cooking a stew after all, and are happy with a quick omelette. Have a plan that's flexible – and I think if you've stocked up on some ingredients that comply with the Method and you understand how to devise a fast meal, it's absolutely fine to plan only about 60 per cent of your main meals. Double up and batch-cook in these early weeks and choose meals for supper that you can spruce up the next day or have cold.

I want to strike the right balance to encourage you to try new meals so you have a range of options that become familiar favourites, without totally bombarding you so that you feel like you're always in food prep mode. I will leave this to you to work out – but the deal is that you DO try new recipes every week. For the first couple of weeks, try the recipes that shout out to you as familiar and easy, and later on you can venture into more adventurous meals to ensure you're trying new flavours and foods because we need to keep it really exciting and satisfying yet always quick, convenient and do-able.

Don't focus on what you can't have – and just bear in mind that all we are doing really is temporarily replacing the heavier carbs with lighter ones in terms of veggies. Focus more on what you're putting in, and not what you're taking out.

As in your Prep Week, my advice is to aim to find two new breakfasts, four new snacks and six new main meals each week – so that you're continually expanding your repertoire.

Most people will find that they end up with a repertoire of about ten breakfasts – perhaps half of those absolute firm favourites – about the same number of snacks and about double that number of main meals, which are interchangeable. Don't forget that all the main meals from all three of my books work with this programme – so use them. But even the meals that become part of your repertoire constantly need changing up.

Whatever you do, don't eat the same meals every week. I have a handful of meals that I repeat often (my Vitality Smoothie, my Vanilla Bircher with various toppings, simple Niçoise salads and an apple and nut butter for my morning snack) but outside a handful of firm favourites, I am always keeping the variety up. Don't let it get stale – it's not nutritious and you'll get bored. Besides, once you've got the principles of the Method and been following it for a little while, you'll be experimenting and adding your own stamp to meals – because really the possibilities are endless.

Do more if you can, but really don't stress if you're experimenting at a slower pace – you have years to try all of the recipes

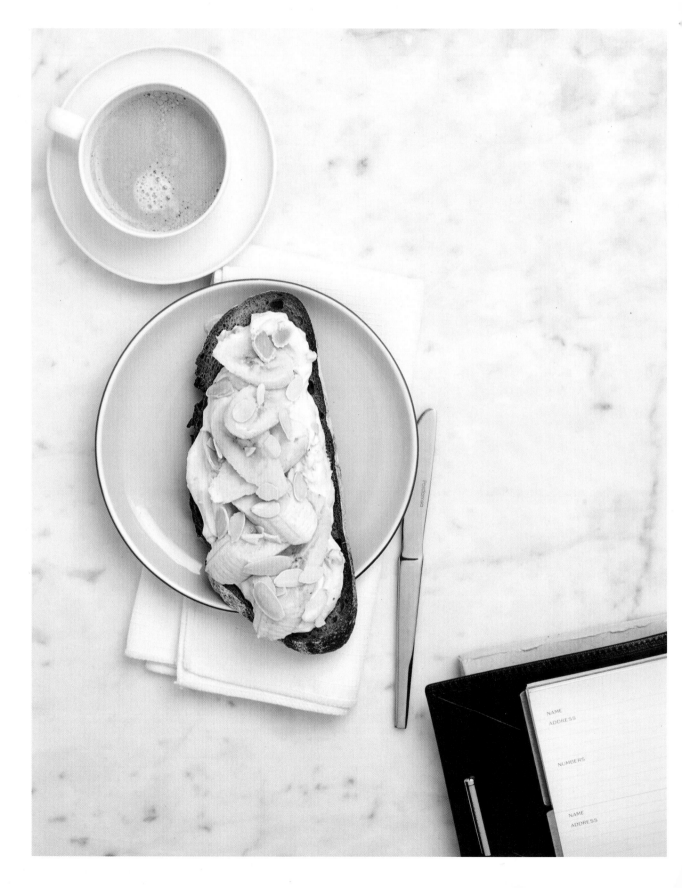

## YOUR FOOD DIARY

I've always spoken about Eating Beautifully more than about eating good, whole, delicious food. Your food should seduce your senses – even if it's just a bowl of porridge in the morning. It's about putting the joy back into food and celebrating your new style of eating in every way possible.

So part of your job is to find the beauty in your meals when you prepare them and present them – to you and your family – and make them a feast for the eyes. I'm not talking about rose petals and carving carrots here – but plate up proudly as it's a sign of self-respect and celebration. An extra minute – that's all – spent on presenting your meals will send signals to your mind that you're eating with joy and you're loving what you eat. Food is meant to be celebrated and if you're skipping the effort, you're subconsciously telling yourself that it's miserable and you're deprived when you're not.

I know the word 'mindful' is overused, but Eating Beautifully really is about being conscious of what you're preparing and fuelling yourself with.

This week, begin to:

- Lay the table for breakfast before going to bed – it'll take five minutes, or you can teach the kids how to do it; you'll wake up to a calmer morning. Eat your meals at a table and never on the go unless you have to.

- Use your crockery, cutlery, place mats and lovely napkins – and don't save wedding gifts for special occasions.

- Serve up your snacks with as much effort as possible – a little side plate, tray and warm drink – and take at least five minutes (you can spare that, phone down) to enjoy it.

- Plate up as you would for guests. Don't overwhelm yourself with portions and use fresh herbs, lemon, lime and garnishes to bring life and zest to your plate. Apply the 'Insta test' – don't serve yourself up anything that you wouldn't be proud for your Insta friends to see.

- In the winter months when you're in need of a PJ sofa supper by the fire, lay out your coffee table prettily and light a few tea lights – just a few minutes marks the meal as a little Pleasure Pop (see page 66) to punctuate your day.

- Never eat standing up or connected to devices. Always sit down and, even if you are at your desk, turn away from the screen for a few moments and take in the meal.

- When you're storing snacks and lunches to enjoy on the go, lean towards foods that travel well so that you're not opening up a soggy mess – invest in containers that are beautiful and that you can reuse time and time again.

- Make ceremony wherever you possibly can – especially if you're trying to revamp how your family eats too. Lovely jars of goodies for sprinkling can turn a bowl of oatbran porridge into a thing of beauty and not gruel.

I advise clients to make a visual food and drink diary in the first few weeks as they kick off. It's so much simpler and more enlightening than counting calories and grams on a food app, which nods to dieting past. Keep it on an Instagram page or the Lean for Life app. Scroll through it at the end of each day, and you can see what's missing instantly. Things to check for:

- Am I trying to Eat Beautifully, with at least some effort and ceremony?

- Are the portions nicely balanced throughout the day?

- Am I getting in three main meals and two snacks?

- How many drinks am I having? Make sure that you're not drinking hidden sugars in lattes, cordials and fruit juices.

- Is my 'Day on a Plate' colourful and varied each day?

- Are there plenty of veggies and is there a good range of different fruit and veg?

- Is there variety? Am I making sure I'm not stuck in a rut?

- Do I feel pleased when I see what I've prepared and eaten over the course of the week?

- What can I improve and where do I need to channel my efforts over the coming weeks?

# WORK OUT INTELLIGENTLY

## INTRODUCTION TO SCULPTING A STRONG, LEAN BODY THROUGH CARDIO-CONDITIONING

I've kept the workouts in this book super-simple and a little bit more classic than my usual approach, as I've focused more on the motions that use multiple large-muscle groups at the same time. I like workouts to be time efficient above all else. If they're snappy and fast-paced, you're far more likely to be consistent with them. And when you begin to see your results improve every fortnight, we take it up a notch. Even with my clients who have personal training with us, we ensure that they have a 20–30-minute bespoke at-home workout that they can do on the move and at home. It's important to learn to train independently, effectively and safely. You'll find a set of five or six moves in each circuit and once you've mastered really good form, I want you to keep the pace up and follow the moves in the order we have designed them, and repeat the set as each fortnight lays out for you. They're designed to give you a total body workout – so that's core (back, abdominals, buttocks, which stabilize your pelvis), upper body and lower body – and, importantly, in a way that keeps you supple and mobile. We're multitasking – each workout will tone your larger muscles and your more delicate muscles and because we're using so many muscles at once – and keeping the pace up – you're going to get a glow on. Conditioning and toning your body with high repetitions using just your bodyweight will also elevate your heart rate throughout. This means your conditioning is doubling up as a cardio workout and so you don't have to drive to a gym and jog on a treadmill. Cardio-conditioning is intelligent exercise – both sculpting and fat burning in one quick session, with the added bonus of elevating your heart rate for up to 24 hours after each workout. The 'afterburn effect' (more officially known as 'excess post-exercise oxygen consumption' or EPOC) is much more pronounced after strength-based sessions compared to steady state cardio alone. This dictates the rate at which your body burns fat after a session. Don't just focus on what you burn in calories during the session; we want to increase afterburn and build a stronger body that burns more calories even when you're resting and drinking a cuppa.

# WORKOUTS WEEK 1

And you're off. Please don't be daunted by the four workouts per week. Each one is really only 30 minutes, and then some mobility and stretching. On days you genuinely have less time, just do whatever you can. I'd rather you worked at consistency over duration (so 4 × 20-minute workouts rather than 2 × 40 minutes) as it's a lot about getting into the habit of pulling on your trainers and rolling out your mat. I find some days they're the hardest moves of all.

So please throw your heart fully into it, even if you've only 20 minutes. As long as you're training the habit to become strong and you're progressing, you'll do just brilliantly.

You've got a circuit routine to practise for a fortnight, before we take it up a notch. I'm being flexible on how many times you will repeat each circuit, as it depends on your time. Don't skip the mobility and stretching; these are just suggestions so feel free to do any of your own moves you know your body needs any given day. You'll likely be familiar with heaps already and check Instagram @louiseparkermethod so I can teach you more as we go.

Begin each workout with the Warm up mobility moves (see page 52). Then spend 60 seconds on each exercise, before moving on to the next. Don't race through them and if you're slowly getting to grips with them, take 90 seconds and have a breather before moving on. The main thing is to focus on your form. Once you're done, flow into the next move. Repeat the circuit until you've spent 30 focused minutes. Finish with your cool down stretches (see page 54).

Pay close attention to your movement; if you're way below 45,000 steps a week, focus on how to bring your count up. Every week, I'm increasing your steps by 5,000, until you reach 70,000. You'll naturally have more active days than others and use the weekends to bring your count up, but remember, the goal isn't to defer all week and play catch-up with marathons at weekends – the aim is consistent daily movement.

**Get into the habit of moving daily – 'paying your daily rent'**

• Get familiar with each cardio-conditioning exercise in Workout 1.

• Aim for four at-home sessions of Workout 1 – up to 40 minutes each

• If you can only do 20–30 minutes, do that. But still aim for four sessions

• Add in any extra mobility and stretches that you know you need

• Walk daily, aiming for a minimum of 45,000 steps spread across the week, more if you can

• Strive, but remember, it's progress not perfection

# WARM UP

## SUMO REACH

1 With a wide stance, point your toes outwards. Slowly bend your knees and bend at the waist to sit down into a seated position leaning forward. Make sure your feet are flat and your knees do not move beyond your big toes. Hold onto your ankles or feet and slowly push your knees outwards.

2 Place one hand inside of your foot and raise the other to the ceiling, opening up your chest. Your head will follow the movement of your arm. Hold for 15–30 seconds, then return to centre position and repeat on other side.

## Ts

1 Start in standing position with feet hip-width apart. Raise one knee to waist height and both arms above your head. Make sure your pelvis is in neutral position and your lower back is not arched. Keep your shoulders relaxed.

2 Keeping your hips square, hinge at the hips like a pendulum. Your arms follow the movement of your hip hinge as you slowly extend your leg backwards. To help with balance, plant the big toe of your standing foot into the floor. Engage your core (pull in your pelvic floor muscles and pull your belly button towards your spine) and reverse the movement to the starting position. Do 15–30 seconds on one leg and then swap to the other leg.

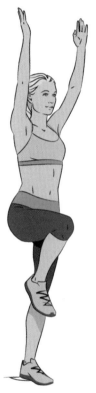

### PROGRESSION

Increase the duration of the stretch

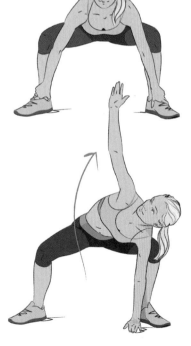

### PROGRESSIONS

Increase the duration of the stretch

Relax the stretch a little as you inhale, and then increase the twist from the torso as you exhale

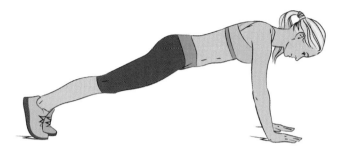

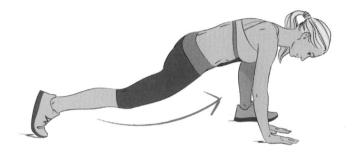

## HIP STRIDERS

1 Start in hand plank position (see page 58) with hands in line with shoulders and a neutral spine (this is where all three natural curves in your spine are in alignment and your posture is good).

2 Keeping your back flat, step your left foot to the outside of your left hand and hold for 10 seconds.

3 Step back to hand plank starting position.

4 Repeat on the right side.

(see page 58)

### PROGRESSION

Once your foot is next to your hand, rotate the arm closest to the foot outwards until it is pointing to the ceiling, following the movement with your head. Hold at the top for 3 seconds.

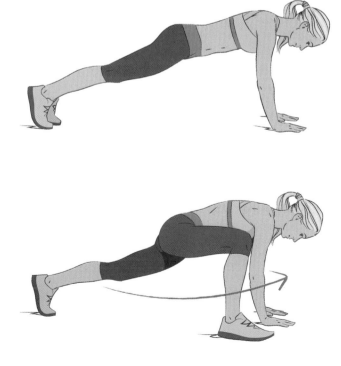

# COOL DOWN

## STATIC GLUTE STRETCH

1 Standing straight with your arms in a prayer position, raise one foot and cross it over your opposite thigh, resting on your other leg above the knee.

2 Slowly sit back until you feel the stretch in your glute. Hold for 15–30 seconds on each leg and swap. To help with balance, you can hold onto a chair if necessary.

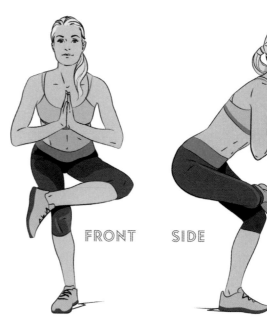

FRONT    SIDE

### PROGRESSIONS

Increase the duration of the stretch

Sit back deeper into the stretch and gently open up the crossed leg from the hip

## CHILD'S POSE

1 Sit back in a kneeling position with feet together and knees slightly apart. Extend your arms out fully, touching the ground in front of you and resting your head on the floor while keeping your bum pressed into your feet.

2 Hold for 30 seconds. You should feel the stretch across your upper back and shoulders.

### PROGRESSION

Take your arms out to the 2 o'clock position. Place your right hand on top of your left hand and relax into child's pose. Repeat on the other side.

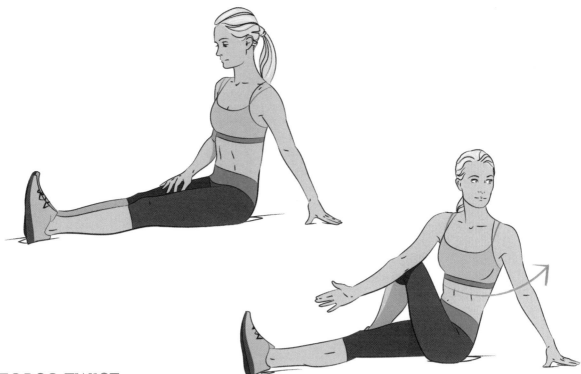

## TORSO TWIST

1. Start in an upright seated position with legs straight.

2. Bring your left foot across your body, planting to the ground outside of your right thigh.

3. Take your right arm, bring it across your body, pushing your left knee away from you while rotating to the left. Your head will follow the movement of the rotation. Hold for 15–30 seconds. Repeat on the other side.

PROGRESSION

Relax the stretch a little as you inhale, and then twist a little further as you exhale

# WORKOUT 1

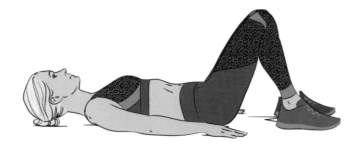

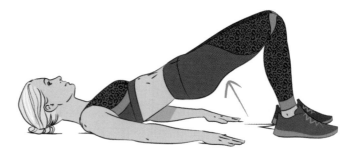

# HIP THRUSTERS

1. Lie down on the floor on your back, with hands by your sides and legs bent. Make sure your toes, knees and hips are aligned.

2. Drive your hips off the ground, making sure you keep your lower back flat. Tilt your pelvis forward, tucking your tailbone in. Focus on activating the glutes and avoid putting pressure on your lower back.

3. Once you have the correct position, squeeze your glutes while your hips are still off the floor, then bring them back down to the ground.

4. Repeat this movement, exhaling while driving the hips up off the ground, and inhaling while lowering the hips.

## PROGRESSIONS

Add mini bands above the knees

———

Add weights on to the hips

———

Increase the repetitions

# HEEL FLICKS

1 Start in a straight standing position with shoulders pushed back and arms by your sides.

2 Maintaining the upright position, raise your left heel off the ground and lift your right heel all the way back to your buttocks, using your arms to balance if necessary.

3 Bring your foot straight back to the floor, then repeat by lifting the left heel. Once you have mastered the correct technique, begin to increase the pace.

PROGRESSIONS

Increase the pace

Increase the time

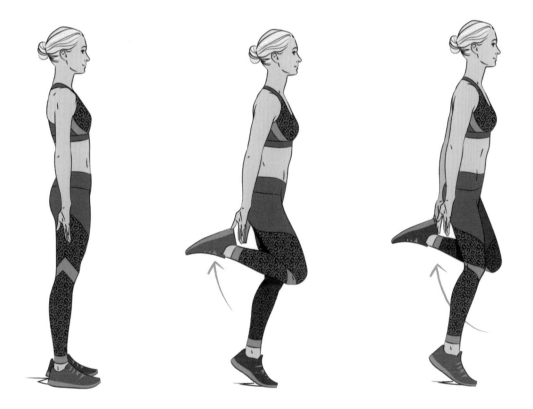

# HAND PLANK

1 Start on all fours with your hands directly below your shoulders and your arms straight.

2 Extend your legs behind you and lift your bodyweight off the ground, keeping a neutral spine with your head facing down to avoid putting pressure on your neck. Tilt your pelvis forward, keeping your lower back flat. Engage your core and squeeze your glutes.

3 Keep your breathing regular as you maintain a strong plank position. Hold for as long as possible while maintaining good form.

## PROGRESSIONS

Hold for a longer period of time

Add small leg raises, one at a time, while keeping your upper body stable

# BIRD DOGS

1 Start on all fours with your hands directly below your shoulders and arms straight. Maintain a 90-degree angle at the knees, keeping them hip-distance apart. Keep a neutral spine with heading facing down and tilt your pelvis forward, keeping your lower back flat.

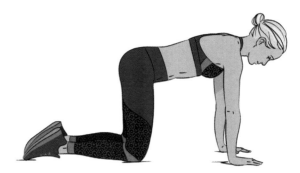

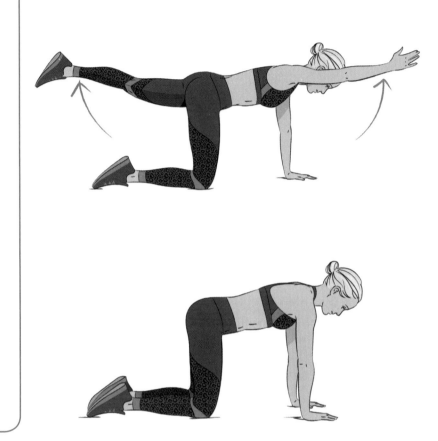

2 Slowly extend your right arm and left leg, keeping them in line with your torso. Hold for 1 second while maintaining a neutral spine.

3 Return to all fours, bringing your shoulders down and back to the resting position.

4 Now extend the left arm and right leg in the same way.

5 Repeat this movement, alternating arms and legs, exhaling while you extend your limbs and inhaling while you return them to the resting position.

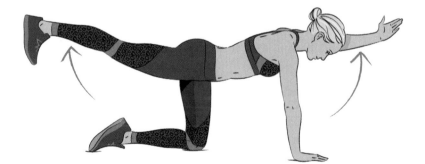

## PROGRESSIONS

Add weights on the ankles

Increase the repetitions

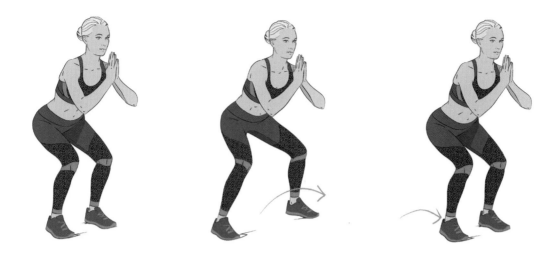

# SQUAT SIDEWALK PULSE

1 Place your feet shoulder-width apart and lower your hips into a squat, making sure your knees do not come in front of your toes. Keep your shoulders back, maintaining a neutral spine, and engage your core. Place your palms together and raise your hands up into a prayer position.

2 Maintaining the squat position, step your left foot sideways away from your right foot, then step your right foot towards your left foot so your feet are shoulder-width apart again.

3 After each step, squat down slightly lower and then return to the original squat height to perform a 'pulse'. Then repeat the sideways movement.

4 Repeat the exercise leading with your left foot and moving in the opposite direction.

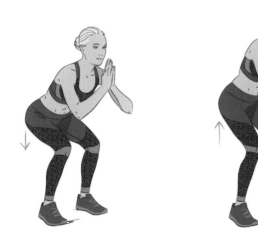

PROGRESSIONS

Increase the repetitions/pulses

Add mini bands below the knees to increase resistance

Lower the squat position

# WEEK 1 CHECKLIST

- [ ] Practise an accountability check once a week.
- [ ] Find a positive Tribe or join #leanietribe #louiseparkermethod.
- [ ] Keep it in this day. Don't project ahead about your doubt in motivation or worry about how tricky it might be tomorrow.
- [ ] Take the routine recce on pages 42–44. Simply know where you're spending your life.
- [ ] Pay close attention to the language you use. Delete the word 'stress' from your vocabulary.
- [ ] Set aside 30 minutes for meal planning.
- [ ] Aim to find two new breakfasts, four new snacks and six new main meals every week.
- [ ] Find the beauty in your meals – spend an extra minute on presentation.
- [ ] Start a visual food diary – check it each day and see what's missing.
- [ ] Get into the habit of moving daily and familiarize yourself with the workouts.
- [ ] Follow the workout points on page 51.

WEEK

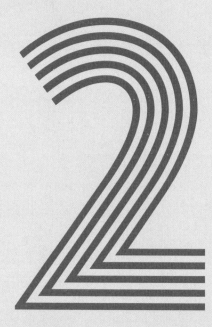

I hope you feel chuffed about what you achieved last week. Please focus on what you have done, and not where you have fallen short. Celebrate each little win, as it really helps build your motivation. If you focus on where you've fallen short, it's really not going to a) work b) be much fun or c) last. You have to do whatever it takes to keep fine-tuning that mental toughness – which is really about having some grit to dig deep in these early weeks in order to practise a new discipline. And turning a negative thought into a positive one as fast as you can. You've got to train your brain just like a muscle and to do this you have to repeatedly catch every negative thought and send it packing. Thinking Successfully is a core part of brain training.

New habits need to be rooted, and it takes time – so you've also got to take a leap of faith and believe that all the effort that you're putting into yourself is going to pay off – a thousand times over. And it really will. Know that you're going to be challenged and decide that you're going to take the challenge head on. Remember that you've only got to discipline yourself and practise mental toughness for so long. Until the habits kick in.

Once your habits are set – and you've results that thrill you – it's just so much easier to keep going. You'll reach a day when you barely have to think about it. Because that's what habits are – just something you do without really thinking about it. Think of the next few weeks as just flipping that switch, to train you to have more of the good habits of health. To become not a health bore but someone who dips into celebration, care free and guilt free, feeling their absolute best.

Do punctuate your day with Pleasure Pops (see page 66) and start to pamper yourself regularly. You're worth looking after. The more you can make your day-to-day a joy, the better. Because the better you feel, the better you take care of yourself and it's all interconnected. Keep finding the joy and pleasure in what you're doing for yourself. Learn from last week, carry it over into this week and just ease into it one week at a time.

# THINK SUCCESSFULLY

## MENTAL TOUGHNESS = ACCEPT THE CHALLENGE

Your body can do just about anything. It's your mind you have to convince. I've met clients and followed the journeys of readers of my books over the years who've overcome just about every challenge there is. You've simply got to know what you want, make your mind up and accept that it's not always going to be a walk in the park, but you'll commit to turning your mindset back round towards success every time you have a stinking day – which you will. There's a difference between saying 'I'll try' and really, really trying.

Everything worth having in life requires effort. What you and I most probably have in common is that sometimes – quite often in fact – we just don't want to work out. Or chop veggies even. And after a period of constant celebration and sitting around, getting started IS hard – nobody finds it easy. It does require effort. What I'm promising is that the effort required to keep going is dramatically teenier than the effort required to get going in the first place.

Accept that it's going to challenge you sometimes in the first weeks until you start getting some reward and return on your effort investment. It's easier to stay up late and skip to the next episode. It's easy to press snooze. It's easy to get into a headspace where you convince yourself you are too old to change. Remember, the challenge is not exclusive to you. If you want the result – the lifelong freedom from dieting and a body that you feel your best in – it's going to take some upfront effort. Make peace with the fact that some of it will be a schlep – but the rewards are going to run over, and God it's so going to be worth it.

But actions that feel hard now, won't always. The effort factor does reduce. Naturally, we want to look after ourselves so much more when we feel better and we're used to doing it. It just becomes what you do, you don't even really stop to think 'Should I, shouldn't I? Can I really be arsed?' and your turnaround time from hesitation and excuse to quick action – the You Turn – gets speedier and automatic. Then the difficulty gap closes and that's a really, really great place to live.

Practise mental toughness on days that challenge you until a natural discipline falls into place. Discipline for most people has to be learned and this isn't about turning you into a bore – quite the opposite. It will eventually give you the freedom to really enjoy life. But like all habits, it takes a bit of time to take hold. Discipline is just another habit, and it needs to be honed. No one's really born with it. Keep practising it and following through. It's literally like a switch and you may have to keep turning it on and off, on and off, on and off until it eventually stays on.

Do the work now, get the habit, get the discipline – and then you can enjoy what's to come (but try to see this process as a pleasure not a chore, or you're just 'stinking thinking' with a mindset of 'only x days to go', again paying lip service to that diet ghost). In time, you'll soon learn the skill of delaying gratification you seek in things that don't bring you closer to your objective right now, so that you can have something staggeringly wonderful in a few weeks time. And remember, it's about delaying gratification over some things, gaining huge gratification over others and still having heaps of gratification when you reach your goal. That's kind of gratifying.

The effort required to keep going is dramatically teenier than the effort required to get going in the first place

# RECOGNIZE YOUR THOUGHT CYCLE

The cycle of change is a mind and body collaboration. I'd love you to become aware of your thoughts so that you can change them. Just note how you're chatting to yourself.

It's not going to happen overnight, but you do need to train your brain, as you will your body. You'll replace negative thinking with winning thinking and it'll take lots of repetitions before you just live in a more positive state of mind. You're going to have down days – but if you want to, you can choose to have more positive than negative thoughts.

For me (and thousands of people we have coached to success) there is a direct link between thoughts and results. It's a simple circle and it all starts with what we think and how quickly we autocorrect our thoughts towards success. It can be as simple as believing that you can succeed.

I know that if a client cannot open their mind to success and change and be willing to see the good more than the ugly, a lasting result may not be possible. It only works if you are genuinely open to it.

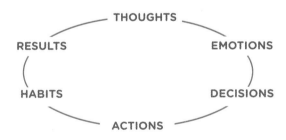

- Your thoughts affect how you feel and your emotional well-being or discontent

- Your emotions then affect the decisions you make

- Your decisions define the next action you chose to take

- Your actions, repeated, become your habits over time

- Your habits directly affect the outcomes of your life

- And what happens in life affects your thoughts

And it repeats – you become what you think about most.

A total head transplant isn't going to happen in a week. You may find that you're a glass-half-full person anyway, you naturally have faith in yourself and are receptive to change. But if you're not, it's going to take awareness, acknowledgment and repeated You Turns in your head. Simply be open to positively improving your frame of mind and keeping an optimistic outlook over the coming weeks.

So, for this week, begin to practise these pointers (I often have to remind myself too):

- Become aware of your thoughts and how they direct this cycle.

- Recognize what you are thinking, when and why – and what causes it to shift positively or negatively throughout the course of your day.

- Notice the power your mindset has over your motivation.

- If you can, take a few moments to jot down the recurring negative thoughts that are standing in your way – you might think 'That's bloody pointless'. Add that to your list.

- Pick up on any thought that will reduce your chances of succeeding at your next action.

- Find a positive counter for the thought, and bring it to mind, even if you're faking it.

- Make sure it's realistic and true to you, something that you can actually get behind and practise.

- Every time unhelpful language pops up, continue to notice it and counter it. Repeat and keep practising it.

- Replace it and practise, practise, practise – even if you don't fully believe it just yet.

A mindset makeover takes time, but step one is recognizing when your thoughts are regularly negative and sabotaging your very next action. Just try – and keep trying to keep a constructive and encouraging outlook on just the next day ahead, not the whole enchilada at this stage. It will all fall into place if you genuinely intend it to.

# LIVE WELL

## PUNCTUATE YOUR DAY WITH PLEASURE POPS

It's imperative we enjoy our daily routine and not just live for holidays and weekends – as this is where we spend most of our lives – so this is a quickie about punctuating your day with little Pleasure Pops. They should be quick and free and screen free. I've no idea what floats your boat, but just start having a think about what little activities and actions in your day lift you up. Simple, old-fashioned Pleasure Pops can just bring about a sense of calm and joy. It's whatever gives you a sense of well-being and contentment – even if just for a few minutes. This isn't about exciting adrenaline pops or necessarily being on cloud nine, but calm and relaxing moments that just induce a sense of tranquillity and real contentedness – a cup of tea under a blanket, a cuddle with your child's warm breath in your ear, a slower walk home than usual. Stress is a weighty issue (no pun intended) and so I urge you to look at any ways you can beat the racing heartbeat throughout the day. Let's look at shoving in some joy so that there's simply less room for worry.

Bring your awareness to enjoying moments of the day that aren't about eating too. If you're not managing to find joy in your day-to-day life, you're naturally going to try to find it at the bottom of a biscuit jar – but that jar will always leave you empty. As you go about your week, pay attention to what makes your heart sing and, basically, do more of what makes you feel good. The more frequent little dopamine hits you can get throughout the day, the easier your appetite is to manage (not to mention you're much more cheerful) and the easier the fight against stress and the release of the hormone cortisol, which plays havoc with your health. So in addition to your brain-naps, just begin to recognize the things that give you the warm fuzzies and do more of them. Note them down and share them with your Tribe. Keep it clean-ish, ladies.

## YOUR ANNUAL HEALTH MOT

If you're busy working and looking after a family, it's so easy to forget appointments and check-ups that keep us in great health. As my life got busier, and I hit my forties, I decided that in my birthday month of March, I would always make sure that I had all the health MOTs in my diary. I usually left them to do 'sometime', and I'd find that over a year had gone by since I'd been to the dentist or had annual check-ups that are crucial to keep tabs on. It's natural to put everyone else first and so I just knew that by batching everything in March, I would always remember in February to spend a morning phoning round and booking myself in for any health checks due that year. I'm not encouraging hypochondria or panic here – but keep a log of when you last had a smear test, mammogram, checked in with your gynae, saw the hygienist and had that dental appointment you've been putting off for months.

I like to make an appointment with my doctor every March to check the basics such as blood pressure and cholesterol, have a blood test if I'm feeling tired for no reason and to just bring up any concerns that have been niggling me but not enough to get round to making a quick doctor's appointment. I spent my childhood in the sun and my twenties sunbathing, and so have an annual skin check too – I'd rather know that all aspects of my health are being regularly checked, as prevention is always better than cure. You'll know what personal aspects of your health need keeping an eye on. Make time for your health and get a system in place so that no niggles or worries go overlooked.

Think too about how you can improve your skincare. I struggle with the time for regular facials but I do try and see an expert at least twice a year – going into summer and winter to help me personalize my skincare routine. I like to see someone who recommends a range of brands and not just their own so that you know your skincare routine is really being prescribed for you.

# MY SKINCARE ROUTINE:

This is my current regime, which I tweak from time to time:

## Mornings

- Quick cleanse with a micellar water, followed by vitamin C serum, hydrating moisturizer with SPF 20–50 and light make-up.

## Evenings

- I double cleanse – first with massage and a cleansing balm and muslin cloth, followed by a glycolic foaming cleanser.

- A couple of times a week I'll use a gentle oscillating facial cleansing brush with my cleanser and follow with a hydrating mask.

- I follow up with a retinol serum (easing off in the summer) and finish with a hydrating night cream.

## For body

- I aim to dry body brush with a natural bristle brush, in long sweeps, towards the lymph nodes, at least twice a week, before a bath or shower.

- Full body exfoliation, using a gentle exfoliator, once a week.

- I love to use magnesium bath salts a couple of nights per week, soaking in essential oils and simple baby bath the rest of the time.

- I use a hydrating body lotion or body oil every single night.

# EAT BEAUTIFULLY

## NEVER GO HUNGRY

I just want to double check that you're not hungry and that you're aligning as much pleasure with your new habits as you can. Check that you're embracing the changes as best you can in your reset. There's a lot of talk about pleasure, I know. But I hope this is the first – and last – health and lifestyle overhaul you'll ever do and for it to stick, it's got to work – it's got to feel good. As we only continue doing what feels good. Simple.

You shouldn't feel hungry on the Method – your meals and portions may be more delicate than usual, but they are spread throughout the day, keeping blood-sugar levels stable and appetite really well managed. And given you're resting and sleeping better – or heading in the direction of achieving that – appetite should be balancing out beautifully.

Equally, don't panic if you get peckish before a meal or snack. You're meant to feel ready for your next meal and it's quite normal to have days when you feel a bit hungrier than usual. You're meant to feel ready, but not famished, for your next meal. If you're genuinely hungry, we need to address it. Check you are not skipping meals and confusing hunger with thirst, boredom or emotions, and that you're getting enough sleep. You can do the Check Five described in Week 5 too (see page 102).

If you're used to having sweets or desserts after meals, bear with it – it's just a familiar habit which we need to make unfamiliar. Try marking the end of your meal with a herbal tea or perhaps a distraction activity such as brushing your teeth will do the trick. Watch out for raw onions and garlic which leave an aftertaste that you often want to cleanse with sweet treats.

The meals are delicate and you're meant to have five a day (three meals, two snacks), just make sure this is the case and you're not skipping breakfast or a snack. If you still feel hungry (or have extra energy needs) you can add in one more snack or increase the size of your protein portion a little. Try to be in tune with what your body actually needs. Make sure you're getting adequate protein and not skimping on the fat – it plays an essential part in making you feel satiated. Try to think about all the plentiful good foods that you are eating – for many it is a much greater volume of whole food – and don't focus on what you're choosing not to eat at the moment. Try not to get your mindset rooted in what you're not having – and focus finding the pleasure in what's on your plate. It's amazing how sweet cherries taste after ditching the 4pm chocolate bar.

Part of never feeling hungry involves seeking pleasure in the recipes. This sounds a really obvious thing to say but it's absolutely vital that you're enjoying the food that you eat. Our job at Louise Parker is to encourage our clients to follow the Method to fit their individual lifestyle, ethnicity and taste buds – and you need to do the same. Don't eat walnuts if you don't like them – swap them with almonds and don't get hung up on simple swaps. Don't force yourself into anything that you simply don't like – but do be open minded to trying new foods.

Make sure that you're happily settling into a new comfort zone by ensuring that you actually find it comforting. Find the pleasure and you'll get that shift. That's the beauty. Fail to do this and you risk saying things like 'I'm starting over on Monday' when you could be eating something you love on Method for supper on Sunday night.

It's absolutely vital that you're enjoying the food that you eat

## HABITS OF HYDRATION

Staying well hydrated can be a real challenge for most – and it's obviously a vital part of your overall health. No amount of water will actually burn fat – but if you are dehydrated, it will slow down the process and, most of all, you'll feel lethargic when we need you to be feeling highly energetic. I know that if I'm dehydrated, I have half the energy levels that I usually do – really don't overlook it.

Everyone has different fluid needs so be guided by your thirst – the optimal amount is very personal to the individual and depends on their weight, activity level, where they live and the quantity of fluids they get from the foods they eat. Just be sensible about it and roughly aim for about 2 litres (3½ pints) a day, including your hot drinks (in which it's sensible to limit the caffeine and milk). Don't go bonkers on water. Excessive water consumption can have dangerous consequences as you can literally flush out your body's essential salts and minerals – so don't drink even water to excess.

Once again, it's just a habit. Once you get into good drinking patterns, you'll find you develop a thirst for more fluids. Ideally you'll be getting most of your fluids from good old-fashioned water, but herbal teas and infusions have just the same benefit. Use common sense and avoid diet drinks and anything with hidden sugars and additives – but the occasional Diet Coke at the pub instead of a half bottle of wine won't kill you either. Remember, we've got to make this work for you in real life.

I don't believe it's humane to take your caffeine from you – but be sensible on it. I drink 500ml (18fl oz) of warm water on rising, then two ginormous cups of tea and one cappuccino if I'm at the office or a meeting. Then I switch to water after noon and generally aim to get in 1 litre (1¾ pints) of water in the morning and the same in the afternoon, slowing down around supper time so I'm not up all night. I find that most people worry about needing to wee the whole time, but turn the hydration up slowly and you'll find your body adjusts.

### HOW TO SNEAK MORE FLUIDS IN:

- Aim to get in about 1 litre (1¾ pints) of water in the morning and the same again in the later part of the day – but listen to your thirst.

- Start your day with 500ml (18fl oz) of warm water, with a little lemon, lime or mint (avoid citrus if you've got gum disease and brush your teeth afterwards). Already you're well hydrated after a long sleep.

- Space out your drinks throughout the day, so that your hydration is nicely balanced. There's no point being a cactus all day and then drowning your body in a big bottle of water which keeps you up at night – space it out.

- Aim for no more than three caffeinated drinks per day, with your last one no later than midday. Two if you can. Any more than three and it'll really start to negatively impact your sleep. Ease down gently if you drink a lot of coffee or you'll have a terrible headache.

- Switch from an all-milk coffee like latte to a small cappuccino and wise up to how much hidden sugar is in your daily coffee – if you're not sure, make your own.

- Chase up your tea or coffee with a little glass of water.

- Avoid diet drinks, cordials and anything containing syrup and hidden sugars. There are heaps of refreshing drink ideas in *Lean for Life: The Cookbook*. Experiment with sparkling water, citrus, mint, passion fruit – it needn't be boring – and learn some good low-sugar mocktails for when you need something yum.

- Avoid too much fizzy water if you're prone to feeling hungry as recent studies say it can stimulate your appetite. But use your common sense, and if it's a case of sharing a bottle of wine with someone or a bottle of sparkling water, you know what to do.

- Keep jugs of water where you can see them and make them pretty. Set up a big jug with cucumber, lime and mint and let it infuse at room temperature. If it's sitting in front of you, you're going to sip away. If it's out of sight, you won't remember until you're thirsty and already dehydrated.

# WORK OUT INTELLIGENTLY

## BEAT YOUR OBSTACLE COURSE

I know that getting the ball rolling with a new exercise regime isn't easy – especially when it's all feeling unfamiliar still and you're trying to work out the best time and the right place to get it done. It really requires discipline and as much routine as you can stick to in the early weeks, before the benefits start kicking in. Equally, if some of the moves are just, well, difficult, it takes a strong will to keep going. We all enjoy doing what we are capable of and are good at – but if it's feeling uncomfortable and hard just stick with it. It's a sign that your body is developing and adapting. It will get easier, and quickly, which is why I'm changing up your workouts every fortnight. I hope you're enjoying your walks and getting outside, whatever the weather. Keep seeing the opportunities in your day to walk instead of drive, or play with the kids instead of sit, and keep looking at what drives the step count up – and do more of it.

On that, if you need to continue with the same workout for a three-week phase, before you feel ready to move on to the next, that's absolutely fine. Work at your own pace, as long as you're putting in your best effort. As a rule, aim to have completed each workout routine at least eight times before you move on to the next. But no harm at all if you do it 12 times, then switch it up a gear.

So well done for getting started and I suspect you've got some aching muscles. Don't forget to take extra time to mobilize and stretch if this is the case. Just a few minutes a day will make a great difference.

We're going to repeat last week's programme, just taking the step count up by 5,000 to a total of 50,000 a week. Please don't panic if you haven't reached that. The main point is that you're genuinely aiming towards it and looking at ways to move more.

I'm sure there have been obstacles – and I hope you've overcome them. If not, don't give yourself a hard time, but do be honest with yourself and work out where the main obstacles were to getting your walks and workouts in.

Now counter them with solutions.

- If it is genuinely a lack of time, you're going to have to go back to your daily planner and make your workouts a priority. Look at what jobs at home you can pass on or do another time so that you have your workout time.

- Recognize where you are 'leaking time' and put an end to those time drains.

- Commit to a regular time for the coming week, in order to build a routine – and set yourself an alarm. When it pings, don't think about it, quick change, create your space and start.

- Keep your workout clothes ready, in a pile and good to go – so you can open a cupboard and your leggings, bra, top, socks, etc. are bundled together for a speedy change.

- If your evenings are really unpredictable, set your alarm an hour earlier in the morning and work out first thing – find one time of day that works for you and stick to it.

- If your steps are falling much shorter than the target, challenge yourself to a realistic number and gradually increase it – but hit your own target this week.

- Don't be disheartened if you've achieved most of it but not all of it. Remember that it is progress and not perfection. If you're feeling demotivated, get someone to join you and make sure that you've a Tribe on board to motivate you. Do whatever you need to do to make it happen.

# WORKOUTS WEEK 2

So, this week, really focus on where the challenges have been – your Obstacle Course – and what you can do to overcome them. Perhaps you need to be tighter on boundaries, ask for help or motivation, be more organized with planning workouts and do all you can to create some You Time.

Once the habit of working out has kicked in, which it will, it is going to get so much easier. Just keep your focus on consistency and really shoot for those four sessions a week, even if you can't put in the full 40 minutes. You may feel that once you've done 20 minutes you actually keep going – this is partly why I would love you to make consistency your focus.

Keep focusing on your precision. Fewer repetitions done with wonderful form are worth heaps more than those that are rushed – so pay attention to the teaching points and keep checking your form in a mirror. No more baggy clothes this week – you need to be able to see yourself properly.

Check in with your movement tracker and keep finding the opportunities to up those steps. We move up to a weekly target of 50,000 this week which I know is not easy. Again, strive for it – but don't berate yourself if you've not hit the golden number. You're still moving more and striving.

**Increase your step count target to a minimum of 50,000 steps this week**

• Another four at-home sessions of Workout 1 – really aim for 40 minutes each this week

• If you struggle with 40 minutes, just ensure you build on last week

• Add in any stretches and listen to what your body needs

• Beat your Obstacle Course – let nothing stand in your way

• Make sure next week's sessions are in your diary

• Have a proper think about how to get your step count up

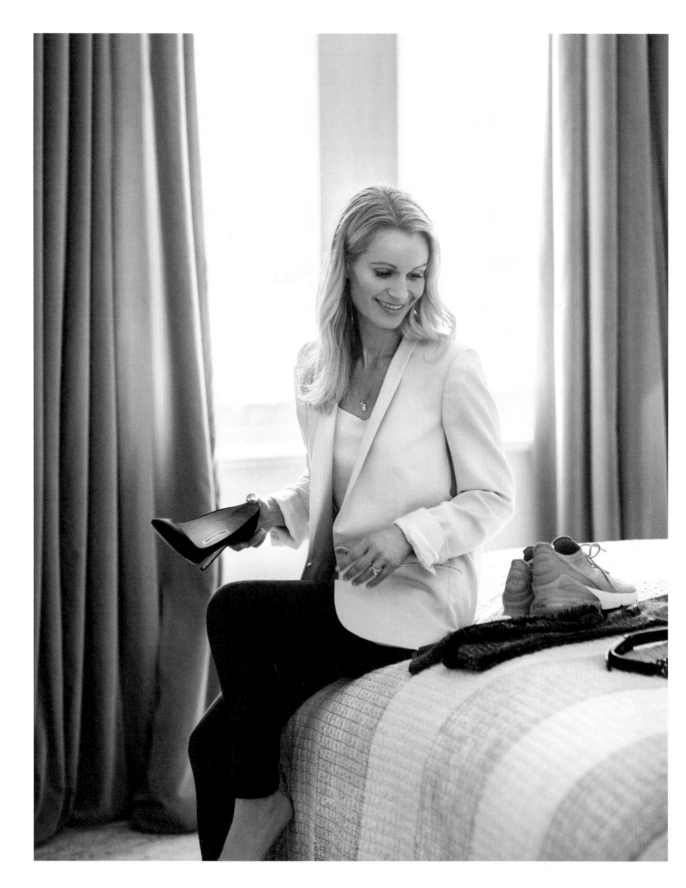

# WEEK 2 CHECKLIST

☐ Practise mental toughness on days that challenge you until a natural discipline falls into place.

☐ Recognize your thought cycle – follow the pointers on page 65.

☐ Add Pleasure Pops to your day. Write down things that bring you joy and share them with your Tribe.

☐ Book in your annual health MOT.

☐ Take look at improving your skincare routine.

☐ Double check that you're not hungry – be in tune with what your body actually needs.

☐ Focus on staying hydrated – follow the tips on page 69.

☐ Review your workout obstacles and tackle them with positive solutions.

☐ Follow the workout points on page 71.

WEEK

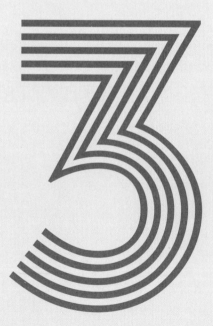

You're a fortnight in and I hope you're taking pleasure in your reset. If not, adjust it – and rethinking your rewards will help. Make sure you're not confining yourself to being home, eating Plain Jane salads and sulking. Get out and have a meal with friends. Just maybe not your Ibiza friends. It's important to learn how to eat on Method out and about and on the go. The principles can be followed in the 'real world', and it's important to see it's not restrictive, and not to overthink it or push a salad around your plate and tell your friends 'I'd love to, but I'm not allowed'. No one likes a diet bore. And all you do is perpetuate this idea that anything transformative and good for you has to be punishing. Remember you will still drink rosé and eat apple tart – this is a temporary phase to reset everything. And I promise, it'll be so worth it.

You're going to learn how to You Turn this week and give up that all-or-nothing mentality, which shreds every type of success. It's part and parcel of learning to be consistent and it will serve you so well later on, when you'll eat and drink with intuition in the Lifestyle Phase.

Tackling stress is easier said than done, but we both know it needs to be done. You won't do it in a week but take stock and lean into the idea that you're going to tackle what's getting to you head on, to make you feel more at peace. You'll feel lighter when you know what has to be dealt with and all is put into perspective.

And without wanting to sound like a West End musical, you're going to Dream a Bigger Dream. I hope you've the excitement and faith to dig a bit deeper. It's so important to have a vision for yourself that's so damn thrilling you won't let anything stand in your way. Best get into the habit now of knowing what you want and being ambitious about it – as we are always evolving. But if you can't see it clearly, how can you move towards it?

# THINK SUCCESSFULLY

## HOW TO YOU TURN

As you know, I loathe dieting. Hate it and hate the 'on it–off it' mindset. It's a vicious trap which keeps you in a whirlwind of setting intentions that are too hard, failing, sabotaging and repeating. But here's the rub. I'm hoping that you find this plan achievable and do-able but know this for sure – you're going to venture off course at some point. Not that I don't have faith in you. But I have been doing this a really long time and I've only ever come across one person in 20 years who's stuck to it religiously. You're going to have turbulence and sulks and your motivation is going to sink. You'll have moments when you're elevated, ecstatic even, as you begin to see and feel whopping change; times when you're just ticking the days off but getting into the groove; and days when you go for dinner at a friend's house with the best of intentions and get home at 3am. Or something along those lines. Perhaps you're struggling to make it work on the go and, while travelling, you oversleep your alarm, get caught short at a business meeting and end up inhaling croissants for breakfast. It happens.

It's oh so tempting – because it may be familiar behaviour to you – to enter into the 'sod it' zone and declare that you're going to start again 'super-strict' on Monday. Or a few days from now, but not at the next meal. And in doing so, what you're actually doing is giving yourself permission to let go and 'start again' full throttle. The problem with this is it keeps you counting days and in a dieting mentality. So you think you're being accountable, but really you're still dieting.

If you eat a burger and fries at lunch, simply choose to eat something on Method at the very next meal. Don't wait a day or three – fifteen meals until you You Turn. When you learn to You Turn swiftly, you learn that The Burger (or whatever) is not the issue. No meal is that much of an issue. What counts are the meals and drinks and moments you have in between what you may perceive as off Method and getting back into the middle of the Method. The Burger becomes just a burger, bowl of pasta, two glasses of wine, cereal in a hurry and so on. The reason

you can get away with eating pretty much whatever you want SOME of the time in the Lifestyle Phase, is because you always You Turn and come back into the inner circle for MOST of the time – so a burger is just a burger.

What makes the Method so easy, and intuitive, is that you have a sleeve full of meals and recipes – whether you're eating at home or out – that are on Method and that you love, so you keep aligning your new habits with pleasure. So it's never a hardship or chore to digest The Burger, then come home and have a bowl of soup and an early night.

So, should a burger pass your lips, don't start moving away from the habits you are building. Appreciate it for what it is, enjoy it, You Turn and crack on. Get your meals back on track – don't compensate and 'go strict' (that would be dieting too) – get your workout in, and still try to get a good night's sleep. I don't even want to refer to it as a 'blip' – and if you perceive it that way, don't. See it as just learning the balancing act of the Lifestyle Phase (which you'll begin to practise in Week 6) and continue with your habits.

People who just intuitively eat well, and maintain their health and weight with ease, do this naturally. Big lunch out, lighter supper. They don't throw the baby out with the bath water. Learning to You Turn until it becomes intuitive could be the difference between you being free or in a diet mentality forever. And no matter what you look like, this still isn't freedom. So please don't panic if you fall short of perfection (which never exists) – do yourself a huge favour and stop sabotaging your forever results with 'starting on Monday' headspace. If you fed a child a burger on a Friday night, you wouldn't dream of filling them with junk until Monday. You'd naturally just balance out what they eat over the weekend. In which case, don't do it to yourself.

So, if you're handed a glass of fizz at a party and neck it, just say to yourself 'You Turn', sod feeling guilty and just keep going.

## DREAM A BIGGER DREAM = SHARE IT

In Prep Week I introduced you to visualizing what you want to achieve. I suspect it felt super-awkward and bizarre. Perhaps you flicked straight past it. It's not easy to be ambitious, which is why most people settle for compromise. But there's a difference between being realistic and compromising what you can achieve.

I'm never surprised that clients achieve so much more than they set out for, but they are continually astonished. I hear 'Oh, I'd be okay with just getting back to a size 16. I need to be realistic' and I'm constantly reminding clients that they *can* reclaim a body that they had decades ago. If you're consistently eating well, training intelligently, living well – what's to stop you? If you're making the journey comfortable, who's to say that you can't stick out the journey?

Is it harder after forty than it is in your twenties? Yes – but not dramatically so. I write this in my forties with peri-menopause and have dozens of clients in their sixties who could give twenty-year-olds a run for their money. We place too much of an excuse on our age. Hormones, metabolism, yada yada – it can still be done. Might take a little longer, but not as long as you think. And if you're on the fence with self-doubt, please just take my word for it.

It's easy to aim for good enough and hard to strive for a bloody fantastic result – where you have a better body than decades ago and are in staggeringly better health. We somehow believe that maintaining an okay body is easier than one that's in rude health, strong and lean as it can be for whatever age you are. Maintenance is just that – it's maintaining what you have. It's no harder to live the Lifestyle Phase in a size 10 body as it is in a size 14. Makes no difference at all. So, knowing that it's going to be no harder to sustain being as hot as you can feel, why not place a more ambitious order now? A visual that is exhilarating is way more likely to motivate you than one that 'will do'. Please, please, aim high. The quality and longevity of your life do depend on it. The fitter you are, the more likely you are to lead a confident, happy, fulfilling life – that's so worth swerving pasta for a few more weeks.

So, knowing that your body is to a certain extent like Play-Doh and you can mould it as much as the framework allows, ask yourself, what is it you really, really want?

- Bring up your lifestyle and your aesthetic visuals again. Especially the lifestyle – that's most important.

- Really spend some time mulling them over – take a few days to think about it if you need to.

- Commit it to paper or illustrate it any way you like – actually make a record of what you're thinking about.

- Plant you – in your new look – into the visual and into this new lifestyle you want to be living with ease.

- Use imagery to represent your new lifestyle – so that when you look at it, you get butterflies. Post it on Instagram, in a private scrap book or use Pinterest.

- Whenever you see an image that represents what you're striving for, add it – until you've got a clear vision board of where you are heading. It should be so clear that when you're standing in a checkout queue lined with chocolate bars, you can transport yourself to the 'Movies of your Mind'.

- Keep returning to it, tweaking it and keep asking yourself if you're aiming high enough.

- Share it with your Tribe and if you're struggling to get it done, find someone on the same path, do it together and make it a laugh.

- Pop a note in your diary (maybe every six weeks) to revisit, revise and revamp it, so it's always current and continually inspiring your next chapter.

Don't skip this even if it feels whacko. You wouldn't skip a business plan on a new venture – and this is a business plan for your health and life. We'd never blush at admitting we use an interior designer or financial advisor – and yet we never really stop to plan what we'd love our day-to-day life to look like. So Ink It, don't just Think It, and keep revising it as we are always work in progress.

# LIVE WELL

## TACKLE STRESS

I spoke about the different kinds of stress in detail in my first book. I categorized them into four types – Lion Stroking (good stress), Mossie Bites (niggles, but you can only cope with so many), Scorpian Bites (bad shocks, but you always survive them) and Shark Attacks (the big issues, which may take months to resolve and destress from).

Simply put, the more we dissolve the niggles and the bigger worries, the easier it is to move forward feeling lighter. We know that stress has a staggeringly detrimental effect on our mental well-being – and demanding lifestyles can prevent us facing it head on. Try to spend a bit of time this week reflecting on what's stressing you out, how best you can take charge of it and let go of it. Know that you will always have a base level of stress – this is about ridding any excess baggage that's weighing you down, physically and mentally. Stress that feels suffocating can be a total hinderance to getting the best result.

I think nothing beats sharing your worries with another – so do this if you can, offload it and get another perspective. But first it helps to recognize what the main worries are so that you can take action and begin to live in the solution and not the problem.

I'd suggest taking no more than 30 minutes to write two lists. Firstly, list only the things that immediately come to mind that are worrying you and causing the most anxiety. If it doesn't come to mind straight away, forget it. List all the niggles, no matter how small they are. Anything that's bugging you and taking up headspace, whack it down. They may be teeny things or they may be bigger hurdles. On the second list, write down all your big worries – the concerns that get you down, cause you anxiety and eat away at your happiness. I'm hoping there aren't too many.

Next up – and be ruthless about this – swipe a line through all the things in both lists that you are powerless over. The stresses that you can do absolutely bugger all about. Realize that you need to let go of anything with a strike-through as best as you possibly can. I know that's a tall order but our time is so wasted worrying about things we cannot change.

Turn your attention to anything remaining on your lists and imagine that you're presenting these worries to your wisest friend. Conjure up that person in your mind – the one who tackles things head on and has a mindset that you really admire. Underneath each point, jot down a few actions that are intended to take you closer to resolving the problem completely or at least reducing it to a really manageable level. They need to be things you can actually physically do – if you can't, they deserve a strike-through.

Now you've got an outline of the actions you need to do in order to deal with any overload of stress in your life. Some might look really uncomfortable, some may take months (but that's okay as you have a plan) and some might require just a five-minute phone call.

Make a note of what you need help with – you needn't do it all alone – then make a note of what you just need to move along as soon as you can. Rewrite your list without the strike-throughs which you can't control, and place each action in order of what you're going to handle first. No need to do it all this week – or month even – but have a plan and make a commitment to do two or three of the action points each week.

Keep it in a notebook in a private place, perhaps your bedside drawer, so that you can add to it should anything be weighing you down – especially at night time before you go to sleep. Once it's written down, you're acknowledging that it's on your list, it won't be forgotten and accept you can't do anything about it now but rest up.

Once you know that you've identified the niggles and real concerns in your current life and you're actively letting go of what you can't control – you're taking action over things that you can change and improve – you know that you're doing all that you can, and it's time to let go of as much tension as possible. This will always be work in progress – it's about practising doing the best you can for yourself and others, and letting go when it's fruitless to worry. You'll feel so much more content when you know that you're tackling things head on, logically and calmly.

We know that stress has a staggeringly detrimental effect on our mental well-being

# RETHINK YOUR REWARDS

It's time to stop thinking of food and booze as a reward or a treat. You might have had to exercise some discipline over a pile of warm croissants, but that's you exercising your discipline until it feels much more familiar to do so. It's not you forgoing treats. Because you will eat croissants again, when and if you decide they're 'worth it' or worthy of you, and when you're at goal and ready to celebrate in balance. Remember that all the while you're thinking of food as a reward, you're reinforcing the fact that (at the moment) certain things are forbidden because you're in a temporary phase of avoiding them. To think of any food as 'forbidden fruit' is just going to make you want it more.

So, let's chalk up a list of things that really do feel like rewards and presents to yourself. I know it's not possible to go and splash out on all of these things in less than two months, but define some bits and bobs that are going to heighten the experience of your reset. You can spread them over a year if need be, but really it's about reframing the whole concept of what's rewarding to you. Maybe it's half an hour to yourself in the morning for a quiet cup of tea, beauty products you love or a weekly blow-dry that really lifts your mood. It could be buying yourself a bunch of flowers or a really lovely set of crockery to help you enjoy the ritual of laying your dinner table.

Remember the circle THOUGHTS – EMOTIONS – DECISIONS – ACTIONS – HABITS – RESULTS – THOUGHTS. Something like crisp new bed linen can play its part. It's a part of your spruced-up bedtime habit (which gives you an extra Pleasure Pop, comforts you, helps you sleep well and you wake up rested with your mindset in a really strong place for the day), therefore bringing you a little step closer to your results – closer

than, say, a croissant would today. It's all connected. As you're going through your week, just have a think about areas of your life and home that could benefit from a touch up to enhance your lifestyle and mood.

Draw up your list as you go about your week, adding anything you feel is within reach and would just lift your mood – from something as simple as a couple of blooms by your bed or new pillowcases, to booking in a regular massage or manicure. Work within your means but don't feel guilty in the slightest about treating yourself to anything that helps make home and work more of a pleasure. Once you've reached a target, make sure that you reward yourself and acknowledge your achievement.

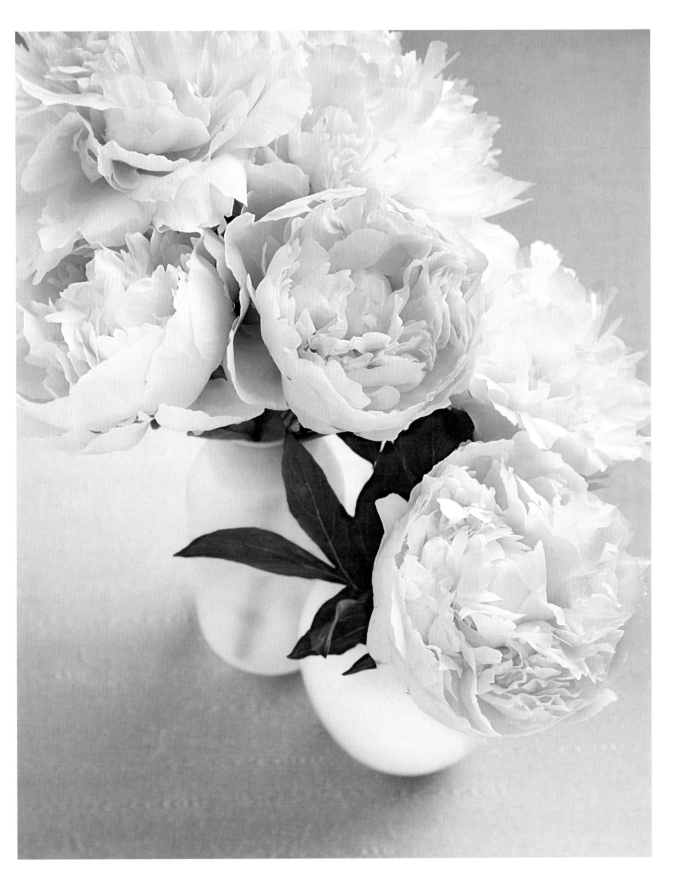

# EAT BEAUTIFULLY

## EATING OUT & ON THE GO

Travelling, eating out and quick fuel stops on the go are likely going to be a learning curve, but embrace the challenge, focus on what you can control and be as relaxed as possible. There are dozens of situations we coach our clients through, until they feel confident and on autopilot when out of their familiar surroundings. Just remember not to set the bar at 'perfection'; be okay with an okay option every now and again, which is far better than not trying. Your only focus is to make the best choices possible in every situation.

It's good to have these challenges as they show you the art of what's possible when you're out and about in normal life and you're motivated, and actually how doable the Method is on the go. You can't restrict yourself to Tupperware or to eating at home forever.

Have a good think ahead to all the situations you have coming up, be they business trips, meals out, busy days without breaks to eat or holidays. And try not to overthink it. Remember some days will be about making better choices, not 'perfect' choices.

In these early weeks, run through the day ahead in your mind knowing where there will be long gaps (very late lunch = good breakfast, pack an extra snack) or meals out (quickly look up the menu for best options until it's just second nature). By navigating yourself through any day that throws you a challenge, you'll learn a lesson and it'll soon feel your New Normal.

My top tip is to squirrel-up and always carry a snack. It needn't be a backpack full but get in the habit of grabbing a bag of pre-prepped nuts and fruit or a protein bar before you leave the house. Make sure your car and desk are stocked and keep it super-simple. Aim for real grub where possible, but protein bars that are less than 5g of net carbs and 20g of protein can sustain you until your next meal. I always carry one on me, along with a bag of nuts.

Restaurants are easier than you think. Have confidence that you know the principles and order like a New Yorker. If you're going to be there hours, have a protein starter and main and skip bread, dessert and booze. These will be back later in the Balance Phase, when they're worth it. Skim through the menu for the main ingredient (a protein) and order any other side or veg that's on Method. If you fancy a steak but it comes with creamy pepper sauce and creamed spinach, just ask for it plain, with an order of veggies and a green salad. Think one protein, a veg or two and a side salad and you're done. Remember that any ingredient on the menu is in the kitchen, so speak out and just ask for what you do want. Don't panic if they've drizzled some butter on your French beans – you've stuck to the principles and that's great.

## DECODING LABELS ON THE GO

Get savvy with food labels and invest some time getting to know what your local options are – both from take-out places near work and your local supermarket. One option could be a ready-prepped bowl of mixed salad. Pick a simple French dressing over anything sweet (or keep your own oil and vinegar at work) and cruise the deli aisle for a good dose of ready-cooked protein – calamari rings, smoked salmon, cooked chicken, prawns or any plain pulses like lentils, chickpeas or edamame beans. Pimp it up with some tomatoes or roasted peppers – keep it interesting and varied. For snacks, fruit and a bag of nuts or a little fresh fruit and a natural yogurt will keep you going – even if it's not the most interesting of meals.

I don't want to bombard you with ideal grams of protein, carbs, fats and fibre and ideal number of calories as really it's about sticking to the principles of protein, low-GI carbs, some fibre and a little fat with most meals. You won't always be on the go, and remind yourself that it's what you do most of the time that matters.

Here are some pointers:

- Aim for a little bit more protein than carbohydrate, but this will vary depending on whether your protein sources are plant- or animal-based. Try to keep sugar content low (below 5g per 100g) and to make sure there's fibre to keep you full for longer.

- Always ask 'Where's the protein?' Protein is key. If you can hit a minimum of 15g at main meals and a minimum of 5g at snack times, that's fabulous. Don't worry if you go over – these are just minimums to try and hit. It'll stabilize your blood-sugar levels and provide damage control when there's some hidden sugar you can't avoid.

- Keep your carbohydrates below 45g at brekkie; and for snacks, lunch and dinner under 20g. If your carbs are from veg, low-GI fruit and fibre-rich foods, even better. Avoid the white stuff wherever you can.

- Keep the fat content below 20g per meal, and ideally stick to good fats. Again, this is just a really rough guide to avoid going coconuts on avocado and eating too many 'natural' and 'healthy' high-fat foods.

- The hidden sugars hide everywhere. Avoid options with 'added sugars', such as fruit concentrate, syrups, honey, agave – but if unavoidable, keep below 10g per meal.

- Shoot for real, whole foods where possible. You can see how processed foods are by the length of their ingredients list – the shorter the better. Ingredients are always written in descending order of quantity, so check it's not a sugar or a fat first up. Saying that, I'd rather have a protein bar on me than fall for a Kit Kat Chunky.

- It's the law to show what is in 100g of a food or meal and so your 300g meal may not be as lean as you think, so don't get caught out by portion size vs 100g. Practise reading labels and eventually you'll be able to eyeball your food and immediately know what the better choice is.

- Calories do matter, but once you've learned how to grab and go, I really don't encourage calorie counting – that's not freedom. If you're completely stuck, aim for approximately 400kcal for a main meal and 200kcals for a snack and you won't wander too far out the circle.

- Make sure you're not drinking your calories – stick to under 200ml (7fl oz) of milk in your coffees and teas and avoid cordials, juices and smoothies without protein – they're packed full of sugar, even if it is natural sugar. If you fancy a fresh juice, aim for a vegetable juice – 150ml (5fl oz) counts as one of your five a day.

- There will be days you might not have time for a proper meal when you're back to back. It's not ideal, but just make sure you're eating little and often. Don't skip meals completely or go hours without eating, or you'll end up with low blood sugars and inhaling the first foods you see.

- Balance the day. There are lighter and heavier recipes in each of my books. They're all on plan and stick to the principles, but we don't obsess about grams and calories – we teach you the knowledge until you intuitively balance things out. So if you've had a heavy lunch, just chose a lighter snack and supper. Your appetite will guide you, so trust it.

- If you're being hosted at someone's home, eat what you're given, balance your portions and relax into it. You can skip wine and dessert but don't phone ahead and be a pain in the arse unless you've an actual allergy. They may not invite you back. Remember this is a lifestyle reset.

- If you're flying, hydrate, eat before you board and bring healthy snacks to graze on. Sleep, rest and eat well on arrival and making sure you sip, sip, sip water throughout the flight.

- Keep going on weekends away and holidays. Trust that you know how to eat off a menu and don't overthink it. Aim for omelette and toast at breakfast, fruit and some almonds for snacks, beautiful seafood and steaks and wonderful local salads and veggies. It really can be done.

- And don't forget to always carry a couple of snacks with you – get into the habit of this and it will really, really help you.

- You will get caught out, but the key is to You Turn and you'll get better and better at grabbing and going. If you end up having a high-carb, high-fat, protein-deficient lunch, it's not the end of the world. You just make sure your next meal is as on Method as possible. Remember it's just a dance – you step back in as soon as you can, and that's a victory in itself.

- In the balance of the week, it all works out.

# WORK OUT INTELLIGENTLY

## TRY ONE NEW ACTIVITY PER
## WEEK FOR THE NEXT THREE WEEKS

This week's challenge is reach out of your comfort zone and commit to trying a new activity each week for the next three weeks. So that's three sessions of exercise that you currently don't do, perhaps have never tried and have been meaning to do for yonks. Book one per week, and try to find sports or classes that you really think you have a good chance of getting into and sustain for a period of time. By Week 6, I'd like you to commit to that activity, once per week for at least three months. Cross-training and challenging your body in as many ways as possible is always a good idea. An overall fitness programme that has a balance of styles of training, encourages the body to adapt and keeps your brain engaged. The programme you're currently following is taking care of the conditioning of all your major muscle groups and you're increasing your cardiovascular function too. I don't want to dictate what you do but see what's available to you locally – and think outside the box. You only need to try one a week – just give it a go and if you loathe it, you never have to return. The purpose is to find a class or sport that you could practise consistently for a good three months. Nothing is off limits – do a PT session or share one if you can, join a run club, try Pilates again, give yoga another breath, pole dance if you so desire – or book that rollerblading lesson that you've been meaning to do for years. (This is actually on my list so that I can join London's Friday Night Skate – so you've permission to kick me up the backside too).

Make sure it's at an hour you could potentially commit to for three months, and importantly that you can afford it. I think if every three months you try a new activity, it's a great way of firing up new skills and adapting your programme to suit the seasons.

# WORKOUTS WEEK 3

I'm hoping by now you've done Workout 1 a total of eight times – and you're ready to take it up a notch into Workout 2.

If you've simply not been able to put the time in, you can repeat Workout 1 for another week or two – it really won't matter if it takes you longer to get to the end of the six weeks of workouts. It's not a race.

Workout 2 gets a bit harder – and you're going to feel the difference. They all progress, but at a sensible level. Stick to 60 seconds on each exercise, but again, if you need longer to get to grips with the moves and your form, increase each exercise to 90 seconds so you're in less of a rush – but still get the reps in. When you get used to them by the end of the week, you can do 60-second bursts next week.

This week I'd love you to add in a new activity – any class or sport will do. You can drop one of your weekly workouts if you simply don't have time – as it's a lot to squeeze in. See how you go. You may find you can fit in five sessions.

Keep checking in with me @louiseparkermethod and post about your progress so the whole community can support you. You'll be blown away by how much encouragement you get from the #leanietribe (set up by these awesome followers who've become great chums following my first book).

Step count is going up a bit too this week. Try to weave it in to your day, so that instead of adding in a designated walk, you're grabbing every opportunity to spread it over the day by walking to work or offering to do the coffee run. Again, progress not perfection. I find it hard to get up to 10,000 a day and it takes time – but try to see it as a game and just enjoy the challenge.

---

**Increase your step count target to 55,000 steps this week – don't panic if you don't hit it, focus on building up gradually**

- Commit to trying a new class or sport

- You start Workout 2 this week, which takes things up a notch

- It's the same system of circuits 4 × per week and keep striving for 40 minutes per session

- Are you still adapting your stretches and paying attention to aches?

- Tweak your diary to make your sessions happen

- Celebrate what you've achieved so far – no being hard on yourself

# WORKOUT 2

## REVERSE LUNGE

1 Start in a standing position with your feet hip-width apart, core switched on.

2 Take a long step back with your right foot and drop your right knee until it is 2.5cm (1 inch) above the ground, maintaining straight hips. Simultaneously raise your right arm and bend at the elbow. Keep your left foot flat on the ground and your left knee directly above your ankle, not forward of your toes.

3 Push through your left foot back to a standing position on your toes and lift your right leg forwards with your knee bent at 90 degrees. Simultaneously drop your right arm and raise your left arm, bent at the elbow. Repeat the exercise on the same leg for 30 seconds then swap legs and repeat on the other side. Always keep your core engaged and hips facing forward.

PROGRESSIONS

Add torso rotation with each lunge, rotating in the same direction as your front foot

Hold weights by your sides or to your chest

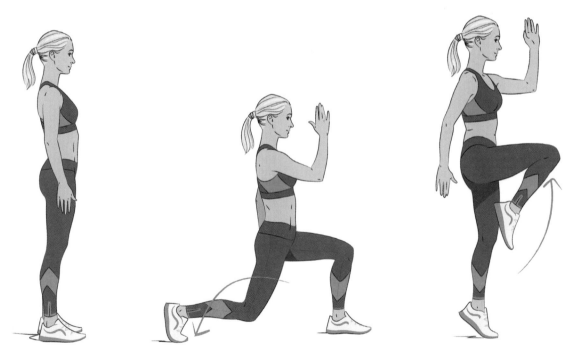

# BEAR CRAWL SHOULDER TAPS

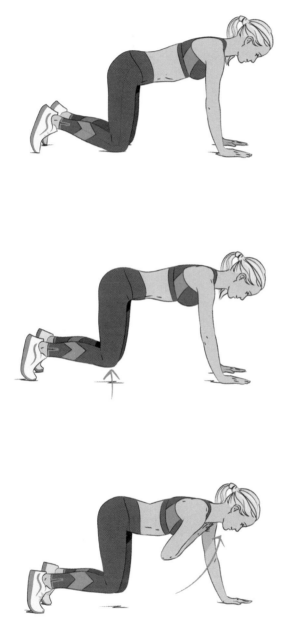

1 Start on all fours with your hands directly below your shoulders and arms straight. Your knees should be hip-width apart and at a 90-degree angle.

2 Maintaining a neutral spine, lift your knees 2.5cm (1 inch) off the ground, engaging your core and keeping your breathing regular. Hold the position, keeping your shoulders and core strong.

3 Tap your left shoulder with your right hand, then return your right hand to the ground. Now tap your right shoulder with your left hand in the same way. Repeat, keeping your knees above the floor, alternating your arms and keeping your body still.

## PROGRESSIONS

Hold for a longer time

Double tap shoulders

# SIDE LUNGE REACH WITH EXTENSION

1 Stand with your feet wide apart and hips pressed back, arms by your sides.

2 Bend your left leg, keeping your right leg straight and core engaged. Reach across to your left foot with both hands together.

3 Extend your left arm upward, opening up your chest. Keep both feet planted to the ground and push off from your left leg back to the starting position. Lunge with your right leg in the same way then repeat the exercise, alternating legs.

PROGRESSIONS

Hold hand weights

Increase repetitions

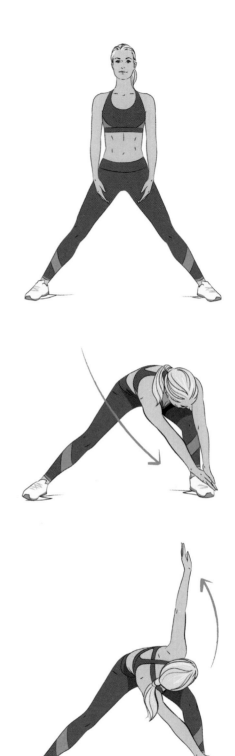

# HIGH KNEES WITH PUNCHES

1 Start in a standing position on tip toes with shoulders pressed back. Raise your fists side by side up to your chest.

2 Drive your right knee off the ground high towards your chest, at the same time punching straight forward with your left arm, then land nice and lightly on your toes.

3 Now lift your left knee towards your chest and punch with your right arm. Repeat the exercise, alternating legs and arms, keeping your breathing regular. It might help to start a steady pace with the legs before beginning to perform the punches.

PROGRESSIONS

Hold hand weights

Increase the repetitions

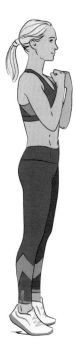
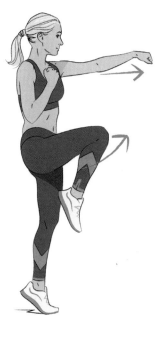
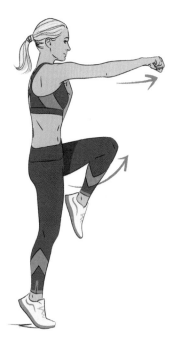

# DEAD BUG

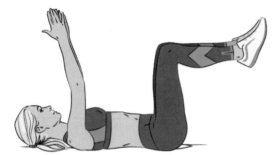

1 Start by lying on your back with your arms extended straight up into the air in front of you. Lift your legs off the ground with your knees at a 90-degree angle. Rotate your pelvis upward, keeping your lower back flat to switch on the correct muscle groups.

2 Slowly extend your left arm and your right leg to the ground while you exhale, then bring them back to the starting position while you inhale. Keep your back flat and your tummy tucked in.

3 Now extend your right arm and left leg in the same way. Repeat this movement, alternating arms and legs.

## PROGRESSIONS

Extend both legs at the same time

Add hand weights

Increase repetitions

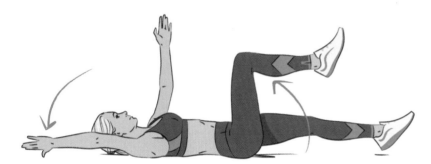

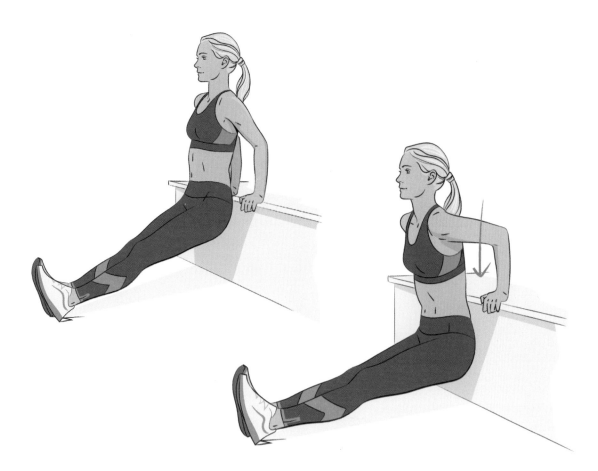

# TRICEPS DIPS

1. Find a chair or a step about 30cm (12 inches) high. Place your hands behind you on the chair or step, shoulder-width apart, with your arms straight and feet out in front of you.

2. Slowly dip down, bending your elbows until they are at a 90-degree angle, then inhale, making sure to push your shoulders back and engage your core.

3. Drive back up, exhale then repeat the movement.

PROGRESSIONS

Place your feet on an elevated box

Increase repetitions

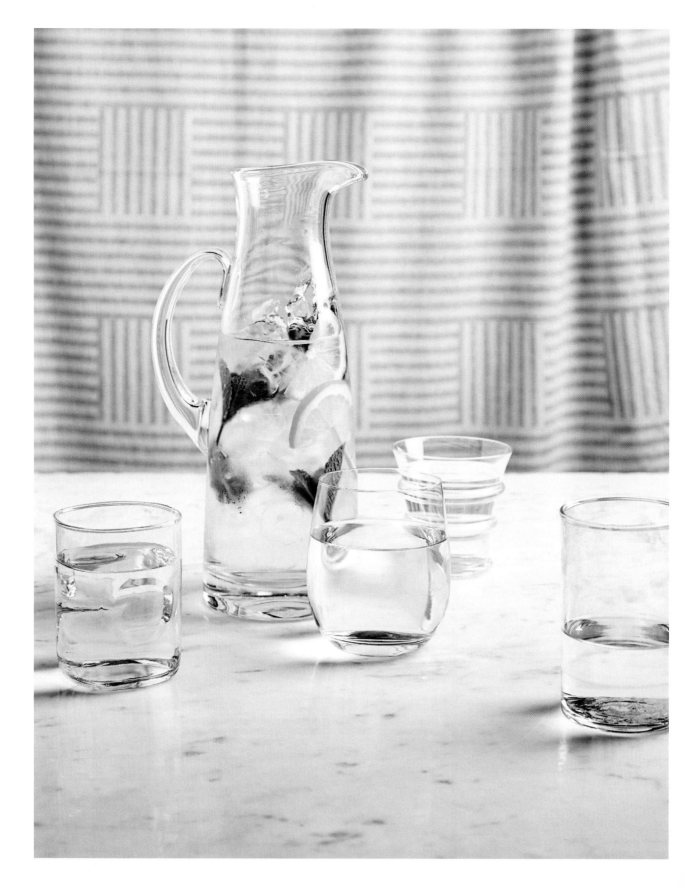

# WEEK 3 CHECKLIST

☐ Remember, a burger is just a burger, so if you find yourself eating something off Method, just You Turn back to the inner circle.

☐ Make sure you're aiming really high. Commit your lifestyle and aesthetic goals to paper and ask yourself if you're aiming high enough.

☐ Make two lists of the things that are stressing you – one of the stresses that immediately come to mind and one of all your big worries. Now strike throughout everything that is completely beyond your control and only focus on tackling those that you do have influence over.

☐ Draw up a list of Live Well elements that enhance your lifestyle and mood. Use them to banish the idea of food and booze as a 'treat' and rethink your rewards.

☐ Think yourself through any days you have coming up where it will be more of a challenge to eat on Method. Remember some days will be about making better choices, not 'perfect choices'.

☐ Learn the principles of building an on Method meal – aim for a little more protein than carb, some fibre and a little fat.

☐ Practise reading food labels so that you can eyeball your food on the go and immediately know what the better choice is.

☐ Try out one new activity this week. Variety encourages the body to adapt and keeps your brain engaged.

☐ Follow the workout points on page 85.

WEEK

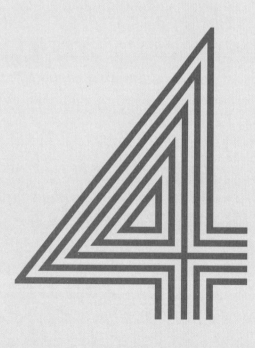

This week you're keeping a check on complacency, working on consistency and making sure you're really training with intention.

Celebrate the strides you've made, making sure you're not chalking off the days. To confuse the two is to say unknowingly that you're not really expecting a forever result. Be aware of that 'nearly done' mentality. Enjoy fine-tuning your day-to-day to create the new lifestyle that you want. Really, really want. The quicker you can close the gap between what is good for you and how you actually want to live, the deeper those habits will be set, the more likely they'll stick – and the greater your long-term results will be. This is the time to really look at anything standing in your way of consistency too, as in this phase, routine is the 'habit glue'. Just until it sticks.

I so hope you start to feel like you've got your groove on, a glow about you and a swagger in your step. Graciously accept every compliment with a 'thank you' and never put yourself down. You've been sleeping and moving more, nourishing yourself with good grub, minimizing stress and reconnecting with muscles that have been snoozing. And the results are going to really start popping soon. Throw that extra energy into this coming week.

The is a big week for Living Well as you kick off a home edit – and as you tick off each room and area of your life, I know your shoulders are going to drop a few inches. Your home should give you a balance of energy and calm – work through it slowly and enjoy it over the coming weeks.

Really watch complacency over the digital detox at bedtime. The habit is so important and it's not an easy one to break. So to stop you loosening the reins, we are going to take the digital detox up a notch this week. Please don't overlook this – it does take discipline, but honestly, you're going to relax so much better and get so much more done without checking your incoming traffic every ten minutes. We coped 20 years ago – so we can do it again for a couple of hours a day. And once you've mastered it, you can tweet about it.

# THINK SUCCESSFULLY

## TRACK YOUR CONSISTENCY = WHATS WOBBLING? HOW CAN YOU BALANCE IT?

Consistency has really tedious connotations, doesn't it? But given so much of our lives are forever moving parts, it can be settling to be consistent and stable in what you do on a daily basis, and repeating behaviours until they feel familiar because we love familiarity. So we're working at aligning everything you do in terms of health with a routine you really feel at ease with. You're less likely to think 'Should I bother?' and just do it anyway.

I'm a firm believer in consistency over severity, every time. Perhaps because I know how beautifully the Method works when you are consistent. We need repetition to glue our habits down. We become what we frequently do, we are a product of how we think every day and our habitual actions.

Perhaps you've tried gruelling regimes before and combusted with boredom or injury. If something is painful, uncomfortable – and I mean consistently miserable – you're never going to get accustomed to it and it probably won't work for you. When we are desperate, we put unsustainable constraints on ourselves. We fail because we're human and humans don't like discomfort every day. This was my pattern and dialogue until I decided to get real, get consistent and avoid dieting and ridiculous unobtainable workout schedules.

I have better results which are a doddle to maintain, heaps more guilt-free celebration time and a much tighter workout regime, now that I've learned to regularly do what works, most of the time. But it took me time to get the habit. The glue is consistency and, again, aligning it with what makes you happy so that you do it with ease.

You're going to do yourself a massive favour if you practise the pillars every day, as habitually as possible. It won't be perfect and if you stumble, just do a quick You Turn and go back to the basics straight away – don't wait 24 hours. The more we repeat what we do, the sooner we are comfortable with it. If it's unsustainable, or really genuinely unachievable for you, examine what needs adjusting so that it is sustainable. It's more important that you find a pace

you can stick at than white knuckle through something for weeks, only to end up feeling defeated.

Once you've got the result you're after, the Method loosens as you introduce the celebrations that you've missed and are worth your while. If you introduce them too soon, you're entering the Lifestyle Phase where you maintain (although you're always evolving) and turn off the 'fat-burning tap' before you're ready. So keep going, be consistent and don't enter the next phase before you're thrilled with your results in the first. Most of all, you've got to give it time to make everything habitual. If you're cruising through the programme, drinking at weekends and missing half your workouts, you're not allowing time for the glue to dry. And that's the biggie. This week, aim to:

- Recognize where you're being consistent and reward yourself for it.

- Notice what habits are wobbling and why, and focus some extra attention to the area that's more of a challenge for you.

- Recognize which areas are harder and ask for help.

- Notice what you're really enjoying and do more of it.

- Ask yourself if you are being accountable. Are you checking in with your Tribe?

- Check you're setting routines firmly in place – waking, workout, meal, digital detox and bed times. Routines route your habits.

- Be patient if you're still relying on discipline – the click will happen. Check you're seeking the pleasure principle.

- Quickly You Turn when you pop out of the inner circle and look forward, not back.

- Make sure you're thinking positively and keeping your long-term visual in the front of your mind.

- Make the programme your own, but use common sense and don't stray from the basic principles.

## WATCH OUT FOR COMPLACENCY & BUST YOUR EXCUSES

The first flutter of anything new is thrilling and exciting – and we have to make sure that you don't get complacent once the honeymoon period is over. The beauty of our programmes is that you have consistent support, motivation and accountability checks. If you're following this programme on your own, you need to notice when you're beginning to drop the effort. Sometimes we don't notice it's happening, loosen the reins too early and confuse it with a plateau. There's great power in momentum and the longer you keep it up, the better the results and the more likely you are to want to stay in the middle of the circle.

Everybody is different but, very generally speaking, you should notice a satisfying step towards results every three weeks you stay consistent. That's truly motivating so take stock and notice and reward yourself wisely for your results so far. Focus on how far you've come and not how far you have to go.

Your consistency check will help this week, but make sure you recognize where you're simply not putting enough passion into your programme, and letting excuses win over, rather than countering them with solutions. While you're hopefully setting routines, make sure you're still mixing up the recipes and trying out your new weekly workouts. Remember to introduce new recipes, be adventurous and ring the changes. Pay special attention to Eating Beautifully this week and don't let yourself slip into sloppy habits. Your body will be adapting now and

working hard and so it's even more important that you're sleeping well and pampering yourself and loving your bedtime routine. Keep finding the pleasure and not the obstacle and it'll keep you leaning forwards.

Don't confuse routine with going through the motions and keep striving to improve. Know that the Method works, that the system is tried and tested – so keep focusing on the Method and hone the habits rather than obsessing about the outcome. Know it's coming your way, but don't make that your sole focus. Keep everything in the day and remember that you're trying to improve your habits every single day. I think if you wake up every day and focus on what you can challenge yourself to do better, with more focused intention, you'll proudly get your head on the pillow tonight and be more likely to try harder again tomorrow. While you've got to notice all the pleasures and benefits coming your way, don't disregard what's challenging and needs your focus to keep moving forward.

Compliments might be trickling in now, which motivates some people to strive and others to sit back – make sure you're not doing the latter. The best is yet to come and so keep it moving. Make sure that you're continually setting yourself challenges (based on your consistency levels you've looked at) to continually progress. Don't overlook anything that you feel is insignificant – like brain-napping and recharging your batteries. Tiredness can kill enthusiasm quickly, so stay alert, revived and keep rewarding yourself at every hurdle.

# LIVE WELL

## DECLUTTER = THE HOME EDIT

Decluttering is the only detoxing that I really believe is actually beneficial to health (unless you're physically withdrawing from drugs). When well fed and looked after, our bodies do a damn good job of ridding themselves of what shouldn't be lingering in them. I'm known to be a bit of a neat freak and cop a lot of flack about it – but I'm pleased to announce that there are psychological studies that actually prove that living in an ordered home and work space puts you at a health advantage, aids concentration and increases the likelihood of you doing regular exercise. So my saying 'A Tidy Home is a Happy Home' is actually fact.

It goes without saying that if everything is in its place – clean and neat – you're instantly going to feel calmer and your stress levels are going to be kept at bay. Add piles of 'stuff' everywhere and your brain is constantly being reminded of all those unanswered letters and chores you haven't tackled yet. I'm not talking about shoving the whole lot in a cupboard (although I do have one of those – and *try* to blitz it once a week, all in one go). Basically, the more visual stimuli your brain is absorbing, the more stress hormones are released – and in turn you're more likely to want a sugar fix and are less able to concentrate on the job in hand.

I'm not for a minute suggesting you need to live in a white minimalist home, but setting time aside to clear out your home is going to help unmuddle your mind, release happy hormones and boost your sense of peace and calm.

Once you've tackled what may feel like a colossal chore, it's just so much less demanding to stay on top of it. Every time you repeat the process, maybe every school term, you'll get quicker at it and have systems in place that make your and your family's life so much simpler.

I'd suggest breaking this down into bite-sized and achievable chunks and enlisting help if you know you're about to tackle a big task. Perhaps you could return the favour to your helper – you'll work through it so much faster and more objectively. Start by walking through your home, room by room, and just jotting down the rooms and the areas that make your heart sink a bit. Start with the hardest jobs first and you'll gather momentum and

enthusiasm as the smugness and satisfaction build. Work out when you're going to tackle each area and set aside specific time too for those areas that weigh heavily on you – like paperwork.

If you've not yet made your bedroom and bathroom your sanctuary – start there and dedicate a day to each. I'd suggest tackling a room a fortnight so that you also have a life. But the trick is to keep the momentum going or you'll just stop after a couple of rooms and be back to square one. Be consistent.

The kitchen is a great place to focus on, as is your dining room – we spend so much time here, especially if you have open-plan living and kids like myself. Make sure the dining table is a designated eating place and declutter that first. A simple vase of flowers or bowl of beautiful fruit will remind you to keep it a sacred space for meal times and conversation.

You can apply this system to every room (and check out all the decluttering blogs and organizational sites which have brilliant storage porn). Empty everything out of cabinets and cupboards and be ruthless in what you keep – think how happy someone is going to be finding your fondue set in a charity shop. Prepare boxes ready for charity shops and blitz as much as you can. If it's not useful or beautiful or really memorable, donate it. Clean out all your storage and put everything you love, need or cherish back in its place. Rejig things around so you feel that things are fresh and renewed.

Make sure your sitting room is peaceful and you have comforts like candles and blankets for chilling out – and banish as many wires and devices as you can. Really embrace a good clean out and use trays and baskets to store everything neatly (perhaps your home workout bits) so that when you're ready to unwind in the evenings and weekends, you instantly feel your shoulders drop.

Don't forget your work space and car – any area of your life that you're spending time in. Take that mental snapshot in your mind and redesign your space to a place of serenity, order and beauty – it'll do wonders for your mood, again aligning your new lifestyle with as much peace and pleasure as possible.

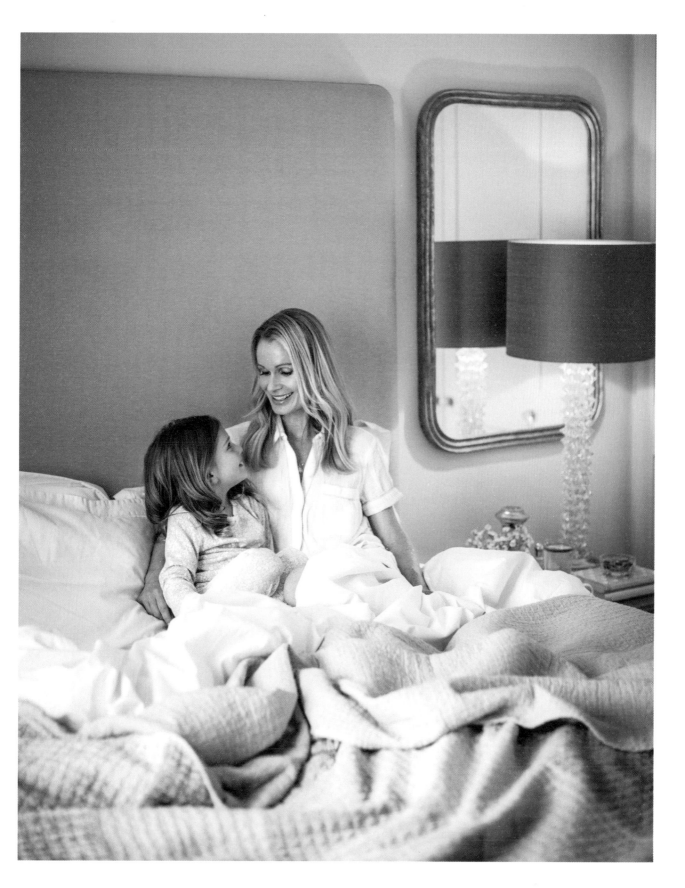

# UNSUBSCRIBE FROM ALL DISTRACTIONS = BE RUTHLESS

Given we are bombarded with so much stimulation – much of it we haven't really opted into, but absorb anyway – this week try to unsubscribe from all distractions, however minute they may seem. A beep of a text alert, the buzz of a WhatsApp chat, constant emails which aren't of any importance and value will punctuate your day hundreds of times. In the effort of the pursuit of more pleasure and less stress, start by unsubscribing to as many emails as you can. Every time you get an email that disturbs your day, unsubscribe from the site. Make a phone call if you know it will save 20 emails back and forth, and avoid getting into the 'Reply All' habit as it's a huge time drain. Unfollow people that make you feel crap about yourself or have values you don't believe in, even if you're curious. Keep your phone on silent and designate certain times to checking it – you'll find that life is a lot calmer if you're not checking your phone every 20 minutes. I find setting time aside in the mornings and afternoons to batch emails and return calls allows me chunks of time during the day to focus undistracted. You'll have a greater sense of achievement at the end of each day – calming down that cortisol. If you're totally addicted to your phone, be utterly ruthless about it and physically turn it off when you're trying to tackle a task.

Last but not least, practise switching off your phone or whacking it in a drawer from the moment you get home for a minimum of two hours. You'll find you relax much more deeply and create mental space to be present with friends, family and meal times. If you can keep this habit going – even if it's just a few nights a week or a half day at the weekend – you'll find that everything quietens down. Within that media stillness, you find so much more delight in the simple pleasures of your day-to-day life.

Keep your phone on silent and designate certain times to checking it – you'll find life is a lot calmer if you're not checking your phone every 20 minutes

# EAT BEAUTIFULLY

## CHECK FIVE

Your results should most definitely be clear now. You should be feeling leaner, your jeans should be feeling looser and your energy levels should be heaps better than when you began. While we are talking about consistency and complacency, there's a little list of five things to double check your eating habits against at the end of each day. They're the basic foundations of the Food Plan succeeding for you and you can't overlook any of them. It's important that you're not dabbling with some of them – they all need to be aligned so that you're well nourished, satisfied and you're firmly in the fat-burning zone.

You have five meals a day and five things to aim for at every meal:

1 **Make sure you're not eating hidden sugars**. One of the most integral parts of the success of the plan is that you're cutting out refined sugars in any form. It's easy when they're in plain sight in white bread and cupcakes but you have to know where they can be lurking. You have a good amount of low-GI carbs in your diet and they're coming from whole sources such as bread in moderation, plenty of vegetables and a moderated amount of low-sugar fruit. Keep educating yourself on where sugar can be hiding or you risk sabotaging your results without knowing it. Many 'natural' foods can have high levels of sugar, so check you're avoiding foods such as honey, agave nectar, 'healthy' snack bars (always check the label for sugar), too much tropical fruit, fruit juices (we always combine fruit with protein and, ideally, a little fat to stop the fructose sugar high), cordials, dried fruit with concentrated amounts of fructose (don't blend dates into smoothies – they're the Haribo of fruit), alcohol and tonic. Just check you're sugar free and tick …

2 **Check your portions are on track – protein and fat in particular**. Keep checking your portions because as the weeks go by, it's easy to get complacent and start doubling up on peanut butter and paying less attention to portions. Bearing in mind that the portions in this plan are not designed precisely for your individual needs; you're going to have to keep paying attention to what feels right and keep an eye on portion slip. It's so easy to get heavy handed with an ingredient because it's on Method. Portions always matter and if you're dramatically swaying from recommended portion sizes, the fat and protein quota could increase detrimentally to feed you more calories than you need – taking you out of a gentle deficit and out of the fat-burning zone. If you're paying less attention to your portions in this part of the programme, it's a good idea to go back to snapshotting your food. Just be sensible, eat more if you need to, but don't start disregarding portion sizes.

3 **Make sure you're eating five times per day – three meals, two snacks**. Eating more delicate portions is only possible because you have smaller gaps between meals and you're eating little and often. You get so used to eating regularly and hopefully your appetite will nudge you to remember to get your snacks in. They're essential to keep your blood-sugar levels stable, stop you feeling ravenous and work towards balancing your hormones. Just triple check that you're not missing snacks – as it will have a knock-on effect on your next meal, which may not satisfy you. Hone in on where or why you're skimping on your meals, turn it around and fix it straight away.

4 **Ensure you're getting a dose of protein at every meal.** Protein has great power for many reasons – and you'll find that there's more in some recipes than in others. For instance, there is more protein in Greek yogurt than in soya yogurt and some sources are richer than others. It's good to have a blend of sources, however, and I don't want you to obsess – everything you need is in the recipes. Just make sure that you're not skimping on protein at any of your meals. Snacks and meals that are adequate in protein are going to fuel your muscle growth, prevent your body burning valuable muscle tissue instead of fat and control your appetite. Start building every meal with protein. Try to pay attention to getting it from a variety of sources – meat, dairy, soya, eggs, beans and fish – it'll help you mix up the recipe variety too.

5 **Check you're including good amounts of fibre throughout the day**. There's an abundance of vegetables and high-fibre foods on the plan and you'll see that any low-GI carbs that are included are always from whole sources. I'm a great fan of oatbran which is super-high in fibre. Enjoy salads, but be careful not to base your meals around leaves only – they won't fill you up enough and you'll find yourself hungry if you're simply eating salad. While I think the salads are delicious, it's important you don't dodge the veggies. Fibre keeps you full, slows down the release of energy into your system and helps your body's waste system to keep you pooping regularly. If someone mentions they're hungry, they're usually not including enough veggies. Pimp salads with crunchy veggies to instantly increase the fibre and fullness factor. I often cook extra in the evenings – making sure they're crisp and kept super-green by plunging them into a bowl of cold water with a few ice cubes after cooking – drain them and keep them in the fridge for throwing into tomorrow's lunch.

Refresh yourself with the details of the Method at the beginning of the book, but use this simple checklist to ensure you're nailing the basic principles. It's simple and you can apply it to meals out and on the go.

## SEVEN NEW SUPPERS & LEFTOVER LOGIC

This week, to avoid complacency, I'd love you to try seven suppers that you've never tried before. Take ten minutes to flick through the books, be open minded and try flavours and foods that you don't usually cook – reach out of your comfort zone. They can be fit, fast food or meals that require more time and effort – but make sure it's all new food that you've not cooked before. Try the meals that don't automatically wink at you and you may surprise yourself. It will energize your commitments and intention to change the way you cook and feed yourself and your family. Perhaps you can prepare a couple of weekday meals over the weekend, so you only have to cook another three on school nights.

It's so easy to get stuck in a meal rut and, while having firm favourites is great, you should continue trying at least four new meals every week over the coming months. You'll have weeks that it isn't always possible – but striving to do that means that you're engaging your commitments and continually finding new meals to love. Only through being open minded and adventurous will you really embrace this varied style of eating.

As you're investing more time in ringing the changes and trying new recipes in the evenings, use some Leftover Logic to make lunchtimes a cinch. Pick meals that can be turned into lovely leftovers for lunch. Not necessarily a cold version of last night's supper, but a meal that you can turn around with just a handful of other ingredients. This is such a good habit to acquire.

I always aim to cook extra on a Sunday, so that Monday's supper (often a comforting chicken soup after a Sunday roast) starts the week off well and with little fuss. Another simple supper is baking salmon in paper parcels with orange, herbs and crunchy veg. I always double up so lunch the following day is a version of salmon Niçoise with leaves, leftover crisp green beans, green olives, a big artichoke heart from a jar, the leftover salmon, a sprinkle of capers and a little French dressing (I always keep a jar topped up – see *The Louise Parker Method: The Cookbook* for my favourites). That's a meal in minutes that you wouldn't turn down at a restaurant. So start experimenting and thinking outside the boundaries of the recipes too this week. If you're avoiding the simple carbs, hidden sugars, watching the fat intake (but not skimping on it) and trying new veggies, you simply can't go wrong. Do your Check Five and trust yourself to experiment and widen your tastes. Most of all, have fun with it and if you're investing more time getting to grips with a new recipe, make that investment flow over into lovely leftovers.

# WORK OUT INTELLIGENTLY

## TRAINING WITH INTENTION

I hope you're encouraged and seeking to find as much enjoyment with your workouts as you can. They're not always going to be a belly laugh and you're not always going to want to do them. You know I promote the idea lof 'Paying your Daily Rent' every day. It's not about gruelling workouts and it's absolutely fine if some days it's as simple as a walk to work or even stretching out your limbs on your bedroom floor for ten minutes – just keep that daily connection to your body. Be aware of ticking off the workouts and putting in the hours without intention – especially if it's a day your heart really isn't in it. Whatever you decide to see through on any given day, make sure that you do it with intention.

You're way better off doing two rounds of a circuit, where your brain is engaged with your muscles, firing the ones that should be firing, than doing four rounds when you're not concentrating and just ticking off the repetitions. It's not about the hours you put in, but the focus and concentration. It might mean that you actually reduce the duration of what you're doing, but hone in sharply to every motion, stretch and movement – and do them very deliberately, with focus and awareness. As you get fitter and more aware of the parts of your body that need more remedial work, more strength, less power and more mobility this will become easier to do. But you'll only connect to what needs your time and effort if you make this absolute connection to what you're doing. If you can, study the movements, seek help from someone more informed that you and keep an eye on your form in a mirror – be totally aware of how you're moving. It sounds peculiar, but as you go through any movement, imagine

planting your brain in the muscles that are working. Use your mind to engage them and to rest the muscles that are meant to be at ease. You'll find it so much more inspiring when you're able to notice the improvements in your fitness by paying close attention to your physical ability, and not just looking for an aesthetic result. Understanding and genuinely feeling what is developing in your overall fitness then helps you to quantify your objectives in the next phase of your training – and keep your regime going with the knowledge that you are always progressing.

Besides your conditioning workouts, pay close attention to how you're walking. Give yourself a posture check, activate your glutes, focus on your stride and be present in any activity at all. The more you pay attention to your movement patterns, bring awareness to them and do them with passion, the greater the benefits – and you'll heighten your enjoyment too.

And the absolute beauty of training with utter intention, is that you get so much more bang for your buck – your results will be accelerated and your time used wisely so that staying fit becomes a habit and not a chore that eats into what feels like most of your downtime. Sometimes less really is more.

# WORKOUTS WEEK 4

Really pay attention to how your body is feeling. You should notice some results kicking in this week, but be patient. You've likely increased your activity hugely, so do notice what might need a good stretch or massage. Perhaps you've got tight calves or hip flexors from all this new movement. As I don't have room to list dozens of stretches that I would have loved to, I'll be posting more for you, so keep me posted with how you're doing on @louiseparkermethod.

Have you started your new activity yet? If it sucked, you can attempt another – just keep trying new things. The goal is to find one you love that balances out the rest of your weekly movement. You may discover a new activity that becomes part of your new life.

This week, try keep the pace up on your circuits, 60 seconds on each exercise, and train with intention. All that means is really focusing on your body, and thinking about what muscles you are using, and making sure that you're executing everything with the best technique you can.

Focus on consistency this week and watch out for complacency – you're half way through your programme and I'm so hoping you're feeling the momentum and motivation build. Do make sure you're checking in with your supporters – it's really important you've others to cheer you on. Pass the support on – helping others can really help heighten your resolve too. Stay accountable to yourself and others and just keep focusing on all the changes you have made.

Step count goes up again too. Don't panic if you're not quite hitting the weekly target – just keep building on it. The main thing is that you are trying, really trying.

**Increase your step count again to 60,000 steps over the week – don't panic if you don't hit it, focus on building up gradually**

- Have you tried a new activity? Switch it if you were just not into it

- Continue with Workout 2 this week and aim for four sessions per week

- If you can only squeeze in three workouts, plus your new activity, that's fine

- Notice what needs stretching and adapt your stretching as you need to

- Tweak your diary to make your sessions happen

- Celebrate what you've achieved so far – no being hard on yourself

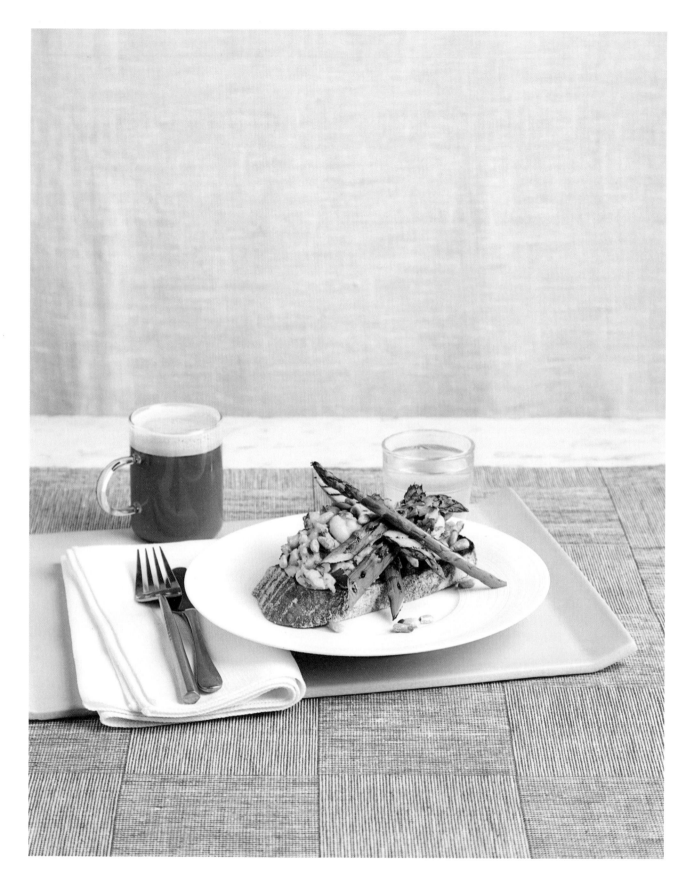

# WEEK 4 CHECKLIST

- [ ] Track your consistency. Recognize where you're being consistent and reward yourself for it, then recognize which areas you are finding harder and focus more attention there.

- [ ] Start your home edit – walk through your home, room by room, and jot down the areas that make your heart sink. Set aside a specific time to tackle each area.

- [ ] Empty everything out of cabinets and cupboards and be ruthless in what you keep.

- [ ] If it's not useful, beautiful or really memorable, send it to the charity shop.

- [ ] Unsubscribe from inessential emails, leave unnecessary WhatsApp groups and unfollow people that don't boost your mood.

- [ ] Switch off your phone or put it in a drawer for a minimum of two hours the moment you get home.

- [ ] Complete your daily Check Five (see pages 102–3).

- [ ] Try seven new suppers that you've never had before. Try meals that don't automatically wink at you and you may surprise yourself.

- [ ] Pay close attention to your posture while walking – activate your glutes and focus on your stride.

- [ ] Try another new activity, or continue with last week's new activity if you really loved it.

- [ ] Follow the workout points on page 105.

WEEK

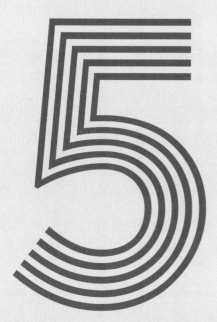

With a month under your belt, you know now that you've got this. Keep bearing in mind that it's all about progress in every pillar of your lifestyle. No one, absolutely no one, does it perfectly. Stay accountable and keep your discipline up. You won't have to rely on it for much longer. I truly think that discipline – like motivation – is a swell that can only last for so long. We do need it to keep the movement going, until everything just clicks and feels more familiar than what you were doing before.

Fast forward five years. As you go about your week, be aware that the habits you're embedding need to last. Not all the time, just most of the time. You'll have so much freedom to let your hair down if 80 per cent of the time you're making healthy decisions on autopilot. Embrace all that you're changing and stay focused. At this point, you don't want to be grasping onto your programme for dear life. If you are, you need to start aligning pleasure and enjoyment with the principles and only you can do that. It's a little switch in the head. Are you doing everything you can to make it a happy plan and simply feel good? Get creative with the recipes and make them your own, get your family and friends on board and go about your programme without declaring you're on 'this new thing'. Keep an eye on your language and try your very best to relax into it.

Your activity levels are really high now, and so do make sure you're resting, sleeping beautifully and getting your brain-naps in. I'd put these things before any other task – make sure you keep your fuel tank topped up.

And celebrate! It's so important to acknowledge how far you've come – don't overlook this. Really enjoy hatching some plans this week to mark your progress and make sure they're properly rewarding – you absolutely deserve it.

# THINK SUCCESSFULLY

## FOSTER THE FIVE-YEAR RULE

With all you've achieved over the last month, and the aspects you still want to hone, it's a really good time to apply the Five-Year Rule. Given we're cultivating lasting change, keep thinking far beyond the next few weeks and months and ask yourself 'Will I still be doing most of this in five years' time?'

Ultimately, the purpose of your reset is for the core of the changes you've made to become the foundation of how you live, for years to come. So as you go through your day-to-day, think about how you can manifest more pleasure into your habits and remember that it's your life to design. Find as much contentment within your week as you can.

Having a routine that's flexible, realistic and ultimately makes you happy will last. But it's dependent on tweaking and really working out how best to adapt it to you – so that it's always aligned with pleasure and not a chore. Ignore that, and you never quite set yourself free.

I'm not suggesting for a minute that you do the same workout for five years or settle into complacency. We need to keep ringing the changes for engagement and progress. It's finding your own pace of doing things, so that you keep going and don't run out of motivation. It's noticing when you're obsessing too much, imploding and starting all over, as you would a 'diet'. That's ignoring the Five-Year Rule. It's remembering that consistency is always more powerful than severity.

It's not about quitting something that is difficult to embed. You're going to have days that truly test your commitment.

Just make sure you're channelling your power into changes that will keep giving back in years to come – and those that make you proud.

Always keep your wits about you, wise up to fads and never put yourself through punishing regimes or 'quick fixes'. I've always maintained that the best sanity check of all is 'Would you be happy if your teenage daughter were to do it?' That rules out quite a lot. Like barely eating two days a week, meal-replacement shakes or anything at all that you know deep down won't survive the test of time and prevents you from letting go of a self-sabotaging 'all or nothing' mentality. Don't mix and match and be tempted to try anything that you know is just absurd, that you know will implode in weeks.

If you have a wobbly week, you swiftly You Turn and just carry on. Keep practising the You Turns until they become second nature. You don't go back to Day 1. Because it's a lifestyle and not a diet. These weeks are here to embed those habits so that in five years' time, you'll just intuitively live a healthier, balanced life.

All the habits you're rooting need to be nurtured and will grow in all sorts of directions which you cannot begin to predict today. You've got to genuinely love the changes you're making, lean into them, celebrate the rewards. Just keep bringing pleasure into everything you can, and even when you're tired and life is throwing you curve balls, your habits will have life. Make sure you're heading towards core change which will stand the test of time – and good sense.

> Think about how you can manifest more pleasure into your habits and remember that it's your life to design

# LIVE WELL

## CELEBRATE PROGRESS

The more you learn to reflect on your progress and celebrate your wins – the more you will have. We simply have to focus on our gains, however small they may be, to keep us motivated and moving forward. Your ultimate visualization may be a while off, and always evolving. We need to stop and really celebrate the habits you are embedding, all the little changes that are binding together to create the future you want for yourself.

Focus on what you have achieved, not what still needs your attention – but don't berate yourself for imperfection. I'm forever reminding clients – and myself – that success is never linear. It's never, ever a straight line from start to finish. There are always dips and obstacles in among the days that seem to fall beautifully into place. Hold yourself accountable, spot the opportunities to keep refining your habits – and try to see them as lessons in what doesn't work for you, rather than 'fails'. Notice how you're speaking to yourself and watch your language – ultimately you're responsible for motivating yourself through days when you feel like just settling for what's easy, familiar – even if that familiar feeling sucked.

This week, make a note of all your accomplishments over the last month. Write freely and don't forget the tiniest triumphs – all the mini changes are conquests too – remember that all the habits, all the pillars are connected and make your transformation stronger. If you've stopped bleating 'I'm so stressed', write it down. If you've started a regular workout of 20 minutes, but it's consistent, write it down. If you've ditched the booze for a month, visualize all those bottles in your head, and write it down.

Time yourself to spend 15 minutes quickly bulleting down all your feats. With speed, freely and not in calligraphy. Just don't put your pen down until you've kept going for 15 whole minutes. It will force you to notice all that you've completed, started, changed or are working towards, and stop you focusing on your shortfalls.

It's not about saying 'Yay, I'm only drinking at weekends' and cracking open the fizz. But just give yourself 15 minutes to really reflect on how far you've come. Please allow it to inspire you – and you simply have to see your progress – as only you can open your eyes to it and choose to notice or ignore it.

Take time to do this weekly, then celebrate your Done It List. When you do, your brain releases dopamine – and you'll be compelled to do more of what makes you feel good and pushes you forward. Share the achievements you're proud of and take pleasure in your rewards. It's a great time to start thinking about revamping your wardrobe, perhaps. What we wear says so much about our confidence – really relish your revamp as you damn well deserve it.

Be mindful about rewarding yourself with something that's going to help you feel great. Remember that food and wine are not 'rewards' – they are just part of celebrating life – and they're coming back in the Balance Phase. It's crucial to break that connection between treats being edible and gluggable – even if they're pleasurable – for you to truly give up a 'dieting' mindset. So, rethink rewards and make sure you're consistently reflecting and congratulating yourself.

# EAT BEAUTIFULLY

## VERY VEGGIE WEEK

My body and health changed rapidly when I decided over a decade ago to eat five smaller meals and snacks a day, balanced with a little protein, fat and low-GI carbohydrates. Protein plays such an important part in appetite control, balancing blood-sugar levels and ensuring that you're not depleting precious muscle mass. However, I don't believe it's healthy, nor balanced, to overload your body with protein – it's simply about ensuring you have a little dose each meal time. Some meals will be higher in protein, some a little less so – but over the course of the week, if you're varying your protein sources, it should balance out.

While meat, fish and dairy products are regular features in the recipes, it's absolutely possible to have success on the Method without having meat at all. Every programme that our dieticians coach at Louise Parker is adapted to the individual client – and we're seeing a huge rise in vegetarian, vegan and 'flexitarian' clients.

Without it being a conscious decision, I've noticed myself cooking far more vegetarian meals for my family over the last couple of years. I've included more vegetarian options in this book – so we now have over 160 vegetarian recipes over my three books.

I'm really conscious of the quality of the ingredients I buy – and I'd much rather invest in well-reared, quality meat and consume less of it, while making up more meals from vegetarian protein. I love good cheese, tofu, lentils and legumes. They're so versatile and if you're trying to eat well on a leaner budget, vegetarian forms of protein are phenomenal at reducing the cost of your weekly shop. Beans and lentils in stews and soups always seem to taste better the next day and are perfect for batch-cooking at the weekend so you have warming meals in minutes the following week. They contain a higher amount of carbs than meat, fish or tofu – so they're good for your higher energy days or feeding a hungry family. They're fantastic store cupboard ingredients and hold well in salads which, if left undressed, last well for tomorrow's lunch box.

I think aiming to eat less meat, and buying the best we can afford, not only forces us to lean into a new style of cooking and try new options, but we play a part in responsible farming and climate change.

This week just be open minded to trying three to four vegetarian recipes and continue to try a couple of options each week with the goal of having a few meat-free meals a week.

# WORK OUT INTELLIGENTLY

## FITNESS WITH FRIENDS & FAMILY

By now I hope 'simply moving more' is coming naturally to you. Your weekly step count has hopefully dramatically increased. Have a think this week about how you can incorporate as many of these steps into active time with your friends and family. If you can catch up with friends over a long walk, instead of drinks, and make it a regular thing, you're just weaving in better habits. You'll find conversation really flows as you walk, just as it would over a G&T.

By being accountable to a pal with a regular meet-up, it's likely that one of you will always feel motivated to encourage the other along. If you can, get a gang of you together to hit some hills or walk somewhere new each week. Encouraging someone who's struggling to get out more will fuel your motivation to keep going. If you can find a handful of good friends to join a workout class with you each week, you're much more likely to turn up and have a laugh. Take it in turns to ring the changes so one of you is responsible for setting the next workout to try. You'll be forced out of your comfort zone and may just discover something new that you absolutely love.

Think of ways that you can have special family time while being active. As devices have taken over our homes, it's so easy to forget the simple pleasures of just being outside, running around with our kids. With no distractions, our bonds can be strengthened by chats you may not have with the TV on in the background. Kids will ask you things that Alexa can't answer and you'll come home feeling fantastic having had a laugh and broken a sweat together. Be the instigator and have someone in the family set the activity for the weekend – and be open to trying something new. Ride bikes together, find a climbing wall, hike, play tennis, learn to skateboard, surf or rollerblade – or simply jog along with the little ones on their scooters. It's about getting outside and doing something new – be open to making a fool of yourself, falling over or getting wet. Without doubt, we all need to be more active as families and so really aim to make a weekend habit of getting outside together – everyone wins.

## WORKOUTS WEEK 5

You're really getting stronger now and I hope you're beginning to feel everything firm up. If the changes feel slow, be patient – they're coming and they're going to astound you. Promise. Keep going.

This week you move up to Workout 3. It's more demanding and you're going to be breaking into a great sweaty mess. The moves have progressed again, so I'd like you to take the first few sessions slowly, paying attention to your form. Form and technique are everything and once you've mastered it, you're going to be able to sustain and progress your results with fast, effective workouts.

**Increase your step count target again to 65,000 steps over the week – don't panic if you don't hit it, focus on building up gradually**

• Move on to Workout 3 this week – focus on form and technique

• Aim for four sessions, even if you can't squeeze in a full 40 minutes each time

• Don't forget to do your extra class – keep searching for one you love

• Notice the parts of your body that need a really good stretch and tend to them

• Embrace a family fitness routine and just get outside and be together

• Make a standing appointment to work out with a friend

• Reward yourself and keep focusing on how far you've come

# WORKOUT 3

## SURRENDER SQUATS

1 Stand with feet shoulder-width apart with a neutral spine. Extend your arms fully up to the ceiling above your head keeping your shoulders relaxed.

2 Slowly sit back into a squat position, pushing your weight down through your heels and keeping your toes, knees and hips aligned. Lower your squat stopping just as your arms begin to move forward making sure you do not arch your back. Explode upwards through your heels, squeezing your glutes and standing tall. Repeat.

PROGRESSION

Pause at the bottom of your squat counting to three before you explode upwards

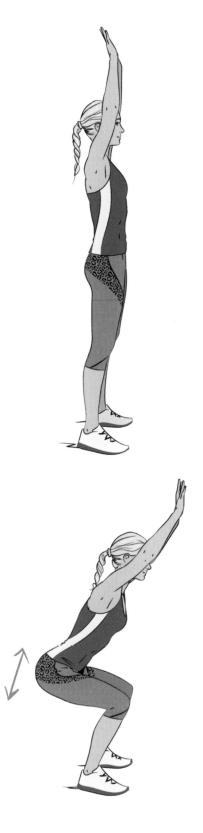

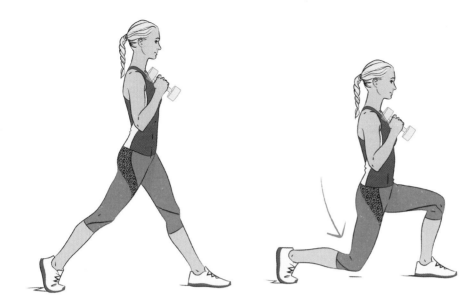

# SPLIT LUNGE PRESS

1 Stand with a neutral spine, both feet facing forward and hip-width apart, holding one dumbbell to each shoulder.

2 With your core engaged and your body nice and strong, drop your back knee down, stopping 2.5cm (1 inch) above the floor.

3 Reach your dumbbells vertically upwards extending both arms fully.

4 Slowly return your dumbbells to their starting position and then, with core and glutes engaged, drive up through your front foot to the starting point. Repeat on the same side for 1 minute then swap legs and repeat.

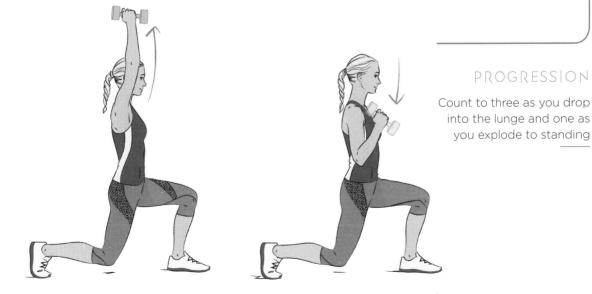

## PROGRESSION

Count to three as you drop into the lunge and one as you explode to standing

# HIPPIES

1 Start on your knees and extend and fully straighten one leg out to the side, planting the heel to the floor.

2 In an upright position, slowly hinge forward at the hips and sit back towards your heel.

3 Drive up, pushing your hips forwards, squeezing your glutes as you return to an upright position. Repeat on one side for 30 seconds, then swap sides and repeat.

## PROGRESSION

When sitting back into your heel, gently twist your torso towards your outstretched leg

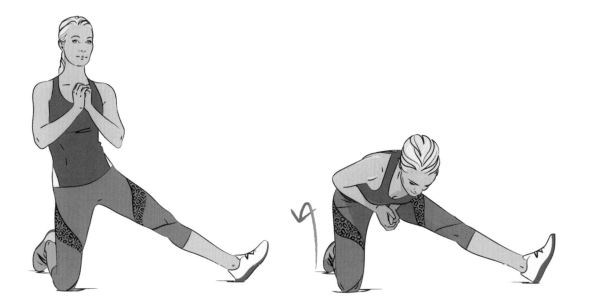

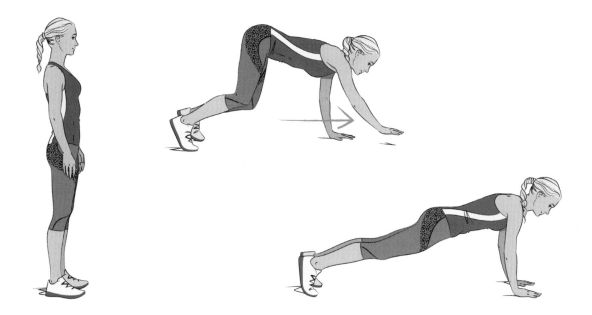

# WALKOUT JUMPS

1 Start in standing position with feet shoulder-width apart.

2 Bend your knees and place your hands on the floor before walking your hands out to hand plank position keeping your tummy tucked in and lower back flat.

3 Hold for 1 second in hand plank position.

4 Walk your hands back to your feet, bending your knees as you go.

5 Making sure you start with your feet flat on the floor, jump upwards using your arms as a lever to explode off the mark. Focus on landing softly then repeat.

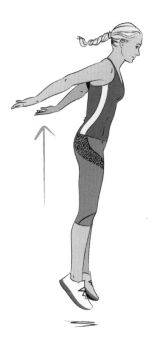

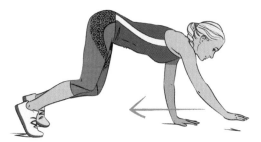

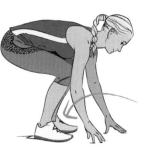

# WONDER ABS

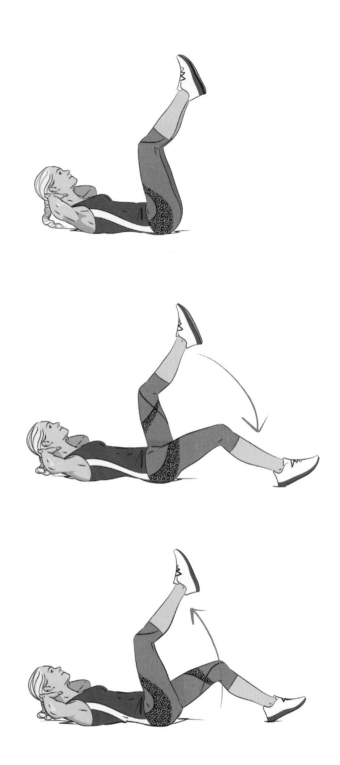

1. Lying on your back, lift your shoulders slightly off the ground, supporting your head with your hands and relaxing your neck. Raise your legs to 90 degrees keeping a slight bend at the knee. Tilt your pelvis forwards so that your lower back is completely flat and your core is engaged throughout the exercise.

2. Slowly lower one leg to the ground while exhaling, gently tapping the floor with your heel and inhale as you return your leg to the starting position. Note the full motion comes from your hip (not your knee) and is stabilized by your core.

3. Switch legs and repeat on the other side.

## PROGRESSIONS

Try to tap the floor silently with your heel, maximizing the control required for each repetition

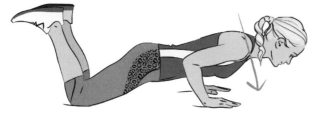

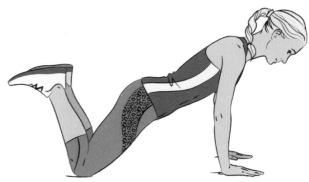

# TRICEP PRESS

1 Start in push-up position with your knees on the floor, arms straight, hands close together in line with your shoulders, neutral spine and lower back flat. Lower your chest to the ground by bending your elbows, keeping them nice and tight to your torso and your back flat. Lower down as close to the ground as is comfortable for you.

2 Drive upwards through your hands and chest, keeping your back straight, returning to the starting position and repeat.

PROGRESSIONS

Pause when your chest is at its lowest point for 3 seconds before driving upwards

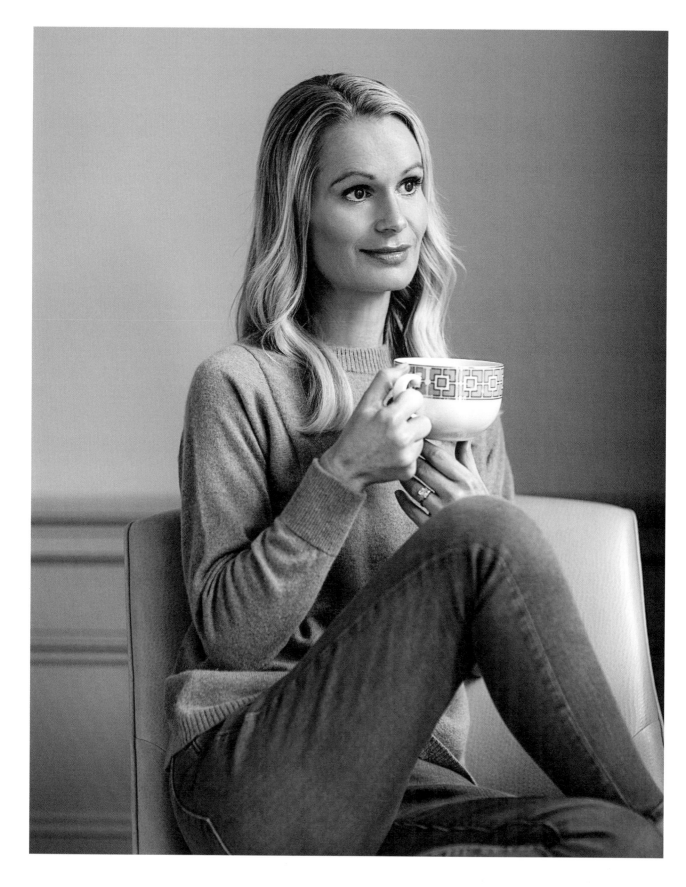

# WEEK 5 CHECKLIST

☐ Look at your habits and ask yourself 'Will I still be doing most of this in five years' time?' Think about how you can manifest more pleasure in your habits.

☐ Celebrate what you've achieved so far! Spend 15 minutes speed-writing down all your accomplishments over the last month, just keep writing constantly until the time is up.

☐ Share the achievements you're proud of and take pleasure in your rewards. Now is a great time to think about revamping your wardrobe, for example.

☐ If you're a meat-eater, try three to four vegetarian recipes this week with the aim to reduce your meat consumption over time. Aim to eat less meat and make the meat you do eat a really good quality.

☐ Think about ways that you can incorporate friends and family into your 'moving more' time. Set a regular date with a friend for a walk or workout class together and make a weekend habit of getting outside with all the family.

☐ Follow the workout points on page 113.

WEEK

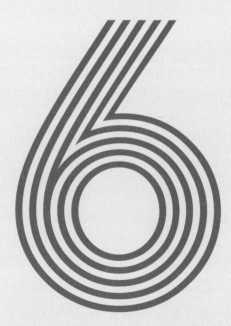

Lean into the last week of your programme with as much enthusiasm as the first. I so hope you choose to do another round and really embed these habits for good. Remember that it's not simply a weight-loss journey – but a path to better health.

Whether you're choosing to do another round to lower your body fat or switching to Lifestyle, do make sure you introduce your 'worth its' this week and enjoy them. Create the habit of enjoying celebrations. Never see food as 'right' or 'wrong' – it's so important to embrace true balance.

My greatest piece of advice as you enter the final week of this reset, is to just keep thinking about your habits and your health. If you keep improving them, your body is going to take care of itself. It'll find its set weight and if you keep progressing your workouts, your fitness and tone are naturally going to progress too.

Keep focusing on the habit and renewing your goals every six weeks, and then one day not long from now, you'll realize that you're just doing it because you want to, in a body that you love. Please check in with me @louiseparkermethod and let me know how you are getting along. Post pictures of your journey and tag me so that I can help to keep you motivated. I would absolutely love to see how you're doing.

Go into this week with excitement and confidence that you've 'got it'. Be aware of what you may need to work on, but don't let obsession get in your way. Remember that the goal is absolute freedom from trend dieting and feeling wonderful in your skin.

Remember not to compare yourself to others – simply strive towards what you know your body needs. I so hope you find the Method gives you a revived, flexible and happy approach to wellness.

# THINK SUCCESSFULLY

## RENEW YOUR GOALS & VISION

I hope you've discovered just how much your body is capable of and are feeling super-proud of your results. Appreciate how far you've come and remember that this is just the beginning. There's so much more you can achieve and strive for, and it's time to renew your goals and plan, and commit to what you want to strive towards over the coming six weeks.

About six weeks into embracing the Method, great things happen. You should be feeling better off in every sense. It's easy to forget how far you've come – appreciate it and build on it. Six weeks is the perfect chunk of time to keep your focus alive and I really recommend that you reset your goals every six weeks – as I do – so you'll never fall into a rut.

This week, take time to reset your goals. Be greedy about them – we have one life and one body. Remember it's not just about aesthetics; if you keep honing the habits, your body will morph into its best. Keep your ambitions high to motivate you, perhaps scare you a little, but ground them in a do-able routine.

Think about the next six weeks as you would a business plan for your body. You're worth that time – don't leave it to chance. While I'm really hoping that habits are embedding, you still need to keep an eye on them, and soon enough they'll fall into place. So for the main part, what you do each day will be intuitive, but it's always time well spent to stop, reflect and revive your plans.

'Think in ink' and write your plans down – and this time round, be sure you're aiming high enough for them to remain as exciting as those in your reset were. Share them with your Tribe and remain accountable – offer to help someone and pass it on – and ask for help from someone whom you admire and who inspires you.

Commit your plans to your diary, just as you did in your Prep Week. Be accountable, share it and keep striving. You have no idea how far you can go, one little six-week chunk at a time. Continue to enjoy it, celebrate your successes, wrap your healthier habits around your family, help someone who is struggling and keep moving forward.

# LIVE WELL

## REFINE YOUR ROUTINE

This task won't take long, but it's worth spending half an hour on. As you enter Week 6 of your reset, look back at your morning and evening routines. So many of our habits are embedded in those first couple of hours after waking and the last few before bed. A day that's kicked off well is bound to set you up well and an evening well spent is going to bring contentment tomorrow.

Think about where you can refine your routine and face up to what's just not working for you. Note it down in half-hour blocks and don't overlook that you may need to slow things down to get more done or ask for help from family. If you're struggling to prepare for your day, fit in your workouts or consistently enjoy your bedtime routine, notice why it's not embedding, what's standing in the way so that you can hone your routine.

While we all have different and demanding obligations, it's fundamental to create a routine that you feel in control of, that bends to each day's demands without leaving you at the bottom of the pile. The beginning and the end of your day are precious – times you want to relish or you'll forever be delaying gratification for weekends and holidays. Keep trying to embed routines and rituals that make you feel good. Shift things around and pass on a chore that helps you get your workout in more consistently. Make sure the workload at home is spread across the family. Keep coming back to this every six weeks, so that you can keep fine-tuning and revising the routine of your own day. It's worth paying attention to the details of your day, so that you can get the absolute best out of it. Make a note in your diary to refine your routine every six weeks or so – or if you have children at school, do this at the start of every half term as I do.

# EAT BEAUTIFULLY

## INTRODUCING 'WORTH ITS'

I'd like you to introduce a couple of 'worth its' this week, even if you're thinking of staying in the Transform Phase and want to continue leaning out. It's so important to be able to introduce a couple of celebrations, learn to You Turn and get straight back to your New Normal. If you're ready to turn the fat-burning tap off, you'll need to start easing into it before you move on to the Balance Phase.

If you've come from a place of dieting it's crucial to learn to let go of that 'all or nothing' or 'I'll start again on Monday' mindset. If you don't see it – and let go of it – it will mean you sell yourself short. And you'll use this plan as a 'dieter' would and never reach true freedom.

So, whatever your plans for the next phase – I would love you to step out a little, celebrate (it's not 'cheating') with meals or drinks that are going to become your 'sometimes foods' and remember that nothing is forbidden. It's time to let go of 'cheat days' and guilt and a good time to re-read the You Turn section (see page 76). Remember, we are what we eat and do most of the time and how we trap ourselves in a habit of 'on and off' mentality is by confusing a 'worth it' celebration as something 'naughty', letting it snowball into eating without mindfulness or intention, and taking 20 days to start eating well again. To break the cycle, it's critical to celebrate, enjoy it and go straight back to your healthy habits.

Think about what you have really, really missed. Note, too, the things you thought you would, but really you don't feel are worthy of you anymore. Eventually this will become intuitive as events and family celebrations pop up, or you decide Friday nights are for fizz and kicking back, or Sunday lunch is a family celebration.

But this week, simply decide on two celebrations which suit your week ahead. Don't go bonkers and keep it delicate – savour and enjoy it. Perhaps you could have a meal out with a friend – a glass of wine, the meal on Method, and share a cheese board or dessert. Or maybe you're looking forward to a comforting bowl of pasta. Make it as delicious as you can, and make sure you have some fibre on the side, a side salad even. If you're having sugar or alcohol, do make sure there's some protein involved as it will lessen the sugar impact and you're more likely to eat or drink delicately. If you bake with the kids, enjoy a good slice of cake – again, maybe after a light protein meal. Don't overthink or panic about what it will be, perhaps wait for the opportunity to arise and just enjoy it.

Do pay attention to how you feel afterwards, as Balance can take a bit of practice. There will be foods that perhaps set you off and that you just find hard to keep delicate – it's usually the more refined sugars for most people – so just make sure that you're never starving hungry beforehand and you're always lined with a bit of protein and fibre.

And if you're continuing on with another round of Transform, simply carry on, having a 'worth it' when you really feel you need it – it's far better for the journey to last longer and feel more sustainable, than for you to be 100 per cent 'on track' all of the time. It may be that you decide to introduce a 'worth it' once a week going forward.

# WORK OUT INTELLIGENTLY

## REFINE YOUR WORKOUT ROUTINE

Right – time to take your workout routine up another notch. This week you're increasing your weekly step count to an impressive 70,000 steps (and if you're not quite there, just keep heading in the right direction).

You're in the habit now of doing your home workouts four times a week and that's a brilliant achievement. Now you're on Week 6, it's time to refresh and change things up a bit. Progression and change is really important to keeping you engaged and continually developing your fitness. You should have a good idea now of what areas you still find a challenge, and what's coming much more easily to you. We tend to do more of what we are good at, and neglect the things we find harder – so just reflect on whether your flexibility and mobility need work and make sure you're spending time on your weakest link.

I hope you continue with the home workouts, and when you feel that you're training with great form and intention and they're beginning to challenge you less, it's time to take them up a notch. You can start to add in variations of the moves that make them harder – but sadly there's only so much I can include in one book. If you follow me on Instagram @louiseparkermethod, I will keep posting new moves for you to follow that you can introduce into your routine.

Your routine doesn't need a total overhaul, it just needs tweaking every six weeks so that complacency doesn't set in. Write down what you'd like to strive to do across an average week – taking on board the new activities that you have tried and enjoyed. Make sure there's a balance of cardio-conditioning home workouts, classes, walking, activities with family and friends. It may be that some of the weekly progressions and suggestions you haven't been able to fit in yet – so have a refresh of them and add them to your workout plan for the next six weeks. What I tend to do is aim to do something every day of the week, and then, because naturally life will get in the way some days, I end up doing four workouts a week. Some will be more challenging, some lighter and some days are just active days with my family – even if that's a long walk before Sunday lunch. Ultimately, when you're in the habit of shooting to do something every day, the habits take hold. And because you're consistent with your workouts, it's fine to have the odd week where you're perhaps paying marginal rent.

Your new lifestyle should feel a pleasure – you do need to keep striving and evolving, but it shouldn't feel an obsession. If you're falling short on what you know you need to do as a baseline, ask for help. Share a personal training session with a friend, do your home workouts with a friend via Skype, anything to keep you accountable. Throughout your week there should be a good balance of what I call high and low days – high days being those with challenging workouts, with easier workouts on the low days and at least a rest day or two. That's not to say you don't move at all on your rest day – always aim for active rest in the form of a walk or bike ride, but do make sure that you're not overtraining too.

If you're living the pillars, you'll be amazed by how your body will continue to develop with consistency and not severity. But always refresh your plan every six weeks, note what needs attention, ask for help when your motivation is flagging and commit your workout plan to paper and the times to your diary. When you look at it, you should feel a sense of challenge but not panic. Set ambitious yet realistic goals.

# WORKOUTS WEEK 6

You should be feeling damn proud of yourself. I hope by now you're really getting into it, loving your new routine and have found a way to set aside this time for yourself. Remember to keep refining your routine – and the more routine your workouts are, the easier it will be to just get the habit of being an active person.

Repeat Workout 3 this week, and I'd love you to end this reset on a really good note. Aim to do absolutely all of it and have a winning week. Turn up for all your workouts. Get out and do your new activity and keep ringing the changes with family fitness. Make sure you've that appointment in the diary to train or walk with a friend. Let's bring it all together. You'll prove to yourself that it is possible and learn what obstacles still need tackling. Then deal with them with lasting solutions.

Think about your next steps and how to keep changing up your workouts over the next six weeks. I hope that I can help you with that. Please keep me posted on your progress on social media @louiseparkermethod as I'd so love to see what you're doing. I'm going to fuel you with new ideas and show you how to keep striving forward.

A word on rest too. Do make sure that you've a day or two a week that you're not doing any strenuous work – walking is absolutely fine. Rest days are really important to allow your body to recover and rebuild. Know when to take it easy and never train when you're unwell or severely tired. Your new active life is to be enjoyed and not endured. It's not about punishing your body or, worst of all, tracking how many calories you've burned. It's about moving more because you love your body.

**Strive to dig deep this week and show up for every workout you can (but do not beat yourself up if you fall short of 'perfection')**

• 4 x 40-minute sessions of Workout 3 and train with intention

• Get your extra class in and your friends and family fitness

• Make sure you are having rest days or 'active rest' days – where you stick to gentle activities such as walking

• Renew your goals for the next six weeks and 'think in ink' – get them down on paper

• Make yourself accountable to someone who motivates you

• Really, really try to hit a total of 70,000 steps this week. Aim for 10,000 per day, but if this doesn't happen, just try to make sure it all balances out in the week.

• Hone that mindset to work out because you are worth the effort

• You're going to have higher activity days and lower activity days in Balance so pay attention to when to strive and when to just survive

• Really, truly celebrate everything you've done and become

• Reward yourself and keep focusing on how far you've come

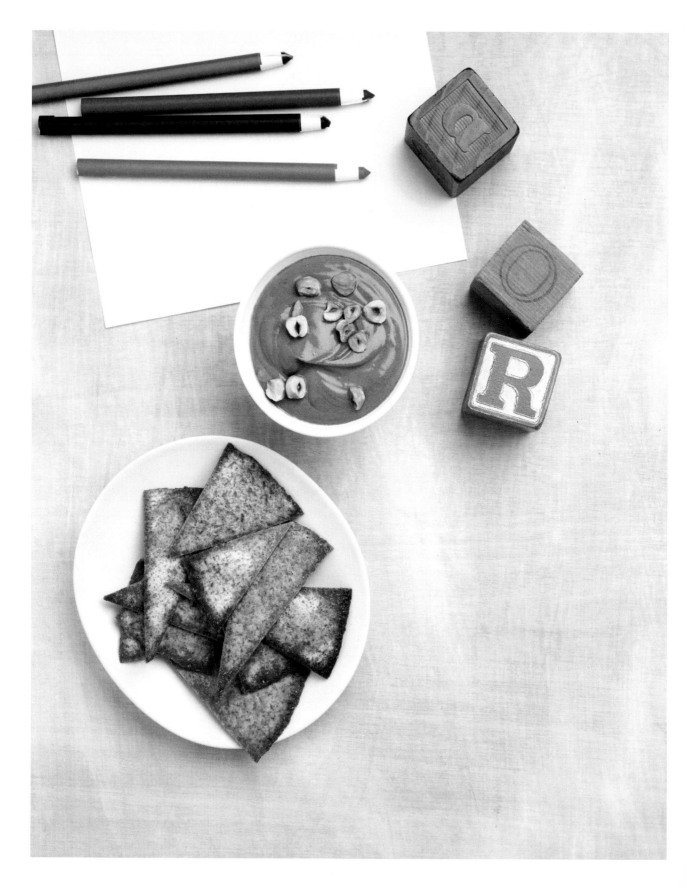

# WEEK 6 CHECKLIST

☐ Start to think about your plans for the next six weeks and think of the next six weeks as you would a business plan for your body. Write your plan down in your diary, be accountable and share it.

☐ Whatever your plans for the next six weeks, introduce a couple of 'worth its' this week.

☐ Look back over your morning and evening routines in half-hour blocks and think about what's just not working for you.

☐ Think about what you have really, really missed and note the things that you thought you would, but really don't feel are worthy of you anymore.

☐ Whatever your 'worth it', enjoy it, and go straight back to your healthy habits. Pay attention to how you feel afterwards – this phase of Balance will take a bit of practice.

☐ Think about the areas that you find more of a challenge and make sure you're spending time on your weakest link.

☐ When you're ready to change up your workouts, follow me on Instagram @louiseparkermethod for new moves that you can introduce to your routine.

☐ Write down what you'd like to do across an average week, taking on board the new activities that you have tried and enjoyed.

☐ Follow the workout points on page 127.

# BALANCE & LIFESTYLE PHASES

## EASE INTO BALANCE

The last six weeks have been about consolidating the habits by trying to be as consistent as possible so that the way you live, move, eat and think should be beginning to feel really familiar to you – with wonderful side-effects that I know you'll find motivate you to keep living this way.

Do as many rounds as you feel you need to, and don't stop before you've got a 'wow' result. Remember that balance and maintenance is just that – it's no harder to maintain a 'wow' result than an 'it'll do' result.

Something kind of magic happens between 6 and 12 weeks and something incredible between 12 and 24 and so if you're still aiming to drop body fat, do keep going. I often see that the results of a 12-week programme can be far more than double the results of a 6-week programme. Don't switch to total Balance until you're proud. You're much more likely to look after a result that's so precious to you than one that's kind of okay.

So simply keep following the Method, loosening it for the odd celebration if you know it's going to be worth it, but in the main, just keep doing what is working. Pay attention to what needs honing and don't become complacent. While perfection is an illusion, assume you're going to aim to put in your best of efforts until you reach your 'wow' and embed habits deeper. I always say the direct route is the easier route and it's a damn sight faster way to get to the Lifestyle Phase, where you'll be following a relaxed 80:20 way of living with a body you love.

You might find that you are ready to turn that fat-burning tap off and that you're as lean as you'd like to be. Perhaps you want to keep working on toning a stronger, fitter body and keep refining your lifestyle. So continue with the Method, keep adapting your workouts and gently transition to an 80:20 way of eating. There's no 'one ratio suits all' as everyone has their own balance – and you need to have faith that you can work this out, slowly and gently and monitoring how your body feels as you do so.

Just remember to ease into it, and don't switch too fast – the natural ability to live this way will eventually click,

but as you begin to add in your 'worth its' do it slowly, thoughtfully and with intention. Try not to overthink it; you will intuitively work out what balances you. Be patient and remember that it may take a little time. You're going to get things wrong, but see it as a lesson and work with it.

Keep bearing in mind that as you're moving closer to your goals – whether that's getting lean, increasing your fitness or creating basic habits of health – your habits are getting stronger. So stay as close to the principles as you can – the longer you spend in the inner circle, with consistency, the quicker the habits will become ingrained. If you keep popping out of the circle you're just not giving your habits a chance to set.

## HOW TO EASE IN & FIND YOUR BALANCE

Our LPM dieticians coach clients individually on how to ease into the Balance Phase and Lifestyle Phase and it's a crucial part of our coaching method. It varies so much more than the Transform Phase. I wish I had more pages to share everything we do – but it's a very personal and individual phase of the Method. I can give you my best pointers and I know that if you pay attention, are patient and trust your instincts, you will get it.

Since I wrote my first book, we've improved the Method (we continually evolve and improve it), separating Balance out as a distinct phase before Lifestyle. We knew from experience how importance the period after weight loss was and the science supports this too. So we introduced a distinct phase where we focus on calibrating the right balance for each client, truly cementing the shift from weight loss to Lifestyle, and creating a simple pathway to follow. Once you've found the balance that works for you, you then shift into Lifestyle, which will feel totally natural because it's your new normal.

So, to switch the 'fat-burning tap' off, you're going to need to introduce more carbs or calories into your weekly food plan. And especially if your workouts really progress and you've a higher metabolism to support. We adjust this for each client and I can only give very general advice here as we haven't met yet. But you've got choices. You can increase the nutritious and high-energy foods such as sweet potato, whole grains including brown rice and quinoa – you get the idea – at all your daily meals. Or you can increase your portion sizes or add in an extra snack.

Let's assume you raise your calorific intake to precisely what your body needs. That's just perfect – you've found total equilibrium, total balance. And if you are balancing your energy requirements and eating the correct foods, you don't gain body fat. However, be aware that when you also add in life's celebrations, beautiful pasta and Pinot with friends, great pizza with the kids, a slice of delicious birthday cake (again, you get the picture), they can tip you into a surplus of energy your body doesn't need – so we switch to slow, gentle weight gain, even if we don't notice it.

Most of our clients continue with the recipes from the Transform Phase, perhaps loosening the reins a little but sticking to the principles, and just ease in, slowly and gently, their 'worth its'. And this creates a perfect Balance. Celebrations are what make the Method sustainable; the couple of glasses of wine on a Friday night, Sunday lunch and all the trimmings – you'll become attuned to what is actually worth it and you'll adapt the Method gradually and thoughtfully. Test the waters to see what makes you feel good, what sustains the body-fat level and lifestyle that you are happy with. If your fitness really evolves, then you may feel you need more fuel day-to-day, so increase the good carbs, or nudge up your portion sizes. And this is how I live it. If I'm home all week, and training hard, I'll simply cook meals slightly higher in energy – and my body tells me that I need it. If I'm out three times a week, I naturally fall back to my usual lower-energy meals when I'm at home and my body kind of tells me I don't need the extra bread.

Now, without knowing what your energy requirements are, what sort of lifestyle you live, there's not a step-by-step plan for finding your Balance. So, you have to trust your judgement. You know that you've got to balance out the celebrations with what you're eating most of the time – and listen to your body. There's no hard-and-fast ten-point plan, but if you get into the habit of eating on Method most of the time, enjoy celebrations some of the time and make sure you really enjoy them – you've found your Balance. Just make the shift a gentle and considered one and pay attention to your body and how you feel. It'll tell you, but you have to listen until it just 'clicks'. Keep practising it, fine-tuning it and it will become your Lifestyle.

## REFLECT EVERY SIX WEEKS

There will always be times that you need to hone in on habits that are slipping – it's a normal part of life to ebb and flow a little. There will always be a pillar that needs a little tending to – whether it's sleep or binge-worthy TV during a tricky time, or noticing when your workouts need more consistency, changing it up and injecting renewed intention. Every six weeks, just take some time to plan, reflect and regroup your thoughts. Keep living well; continue finding pleasure in your morning and evening routines as living well has a profound impact on our mood and motivation. When you keep a close eye on all the pillars and keep paying your daily rent to them, they will hold up your good eating habits. In time, it will be a gentle eye and an almost automatic shift. If sustaining a balanced, mindful eating routine is the harder pillar for you, I really urge you to pay attention to the other three pillars – don't just hone in on the food. Remember how everything is interlinked.

And please don't worry about how long it will take you to find your Balance. It'll be a lot less than the time you've spent trying to find something that works for you forever. So as you reflect every few weeks, try to stop yourself counting and chalking off the days in between. Catch yourself whenever you're falling back into a 'dieting mindset'. You shouldn't need to chalk off anything that you're enjoying and when you're living with ease. If you're 'chalking' Day 32, you've got to do the work that aligns your new lifestyle with more pleasure (as repetitive as I sound). Adjust it, make it sustainable for you. That's the sweet spot, as when you're in this zone of living well and actually loving it, it will last a lifetime and keep giving back to you. So pay attention as you head into Balance with the objective to reach a day where you just get on with it without overthinking – that's the beauty of the habit.

## CREATE YOUR OWN RECIPES

In the Balance Phase, no meal or recipe is off the table. It may be a 'sometimes' recipe, but it's important not to eliminate any foods from your diet forever – you'll only want it more and, besides, I'm wanting a truly balanced, joyful and sustainable way of eating for you long term.

Please think outside the LPM books – look to other cookery authors and learn how to adapt a recipe to make it work to the Method. It's a good skill to know how to pick up a cookbook, and tweak it to the Method so that it can be an 'always' recipe. You know that you want to maintain a dose of protein, plenty of veggies and a little bit of fat. Make sure carbs are low GI and sugars aren't lurking where you can't see them.

Keep ringing the changes and try to adapt or invent a new recipe at least once a week. It could be a super-simple variation of a bircher, a soup, stew or stir-fry – but the best way to really embrace a new style of cooking and eating is with your own experiments. Make sure you share them with us on Instagram – pass the goodness on!

## FITTING IN FAMILY & FRIENDS

I wholeheartedly recommend weaving the Method's principles into family life. Everyone will benefit from eating better, being more active, spending less time looking at screens and getting more sleep. Just do your thing, try not to preach and your family will benefit as if by osmosis.

The recipes and principles of the Food Plan can easily be adapted to allow for growing children, hungry teens and partners with greater energy requirements than you. Whenever possible, cook the same meal for the whole family and make your own adaptations – it's easily done. If you consider the basic principles of this way of eating, it's really just about portion control (which can be adjusted), cooking with whole foods as much as possible (unarguably good for all) and reducing refined sugar intake.

In the Transform Phase – all the recipes across all three books – you'll see that the main meals are lower in carbohydrates. So, all I do if I need to top up the energy content of a meal is add in a delicate portion of good-quality carbs. There's a section in my second book *Lean for Life: The Cookbook* called Extra Energy Sides which includes some of our family favourites.

I hope to raise children who understand that there are 'sometimes foods' and 'always foods' and that nothing is off limits. Real, whole foods most of the time, and not denying ourselves anything. I never refer to a food as 'healthy' or 'unhealthy' as I believe a healthy diet is about a balance of foods. I think we have to be careful about projecting any sort of preoccupation with food (and I hope this frees you of it) onto our children. So while I devote time to cooking, I also balance it with quick assembly jobs, ordering in and eating out. I passionately believe an 'obsessively healthy' diet all of the time is just not normal – orthorexia is a dangerous eating disorder where the sufferer will only eat what they perceive to be 'super-healthy' and don't allow any 'unhealthy' or 'sometimes' foods. So please, celebrate food – don't be afraid of it, never refer to it as a 'sin' or 'cheat' or 'naughty'. All these words linger in little minds that absorb everything they hear.

There's another section in *Lean for Life: The Cookbook*, Good Enough for Guests, that contains recipes for entertaining – but essentially if I'm hosting I'll simply cook whatever I fancy and enjoy it. If you're cooking for friends and you're still in your reset, you'll be surprised how happy they will be with dozens of the recipes. Plonk a lovely basket of bread and butter on the table, some good wine and you're good to go. And if you're hosting Sunday lunch in your reset, simply keep your portion a bit more delicate and maybe avoid the roast potatoes. In the Balance Phase you'll enjoy these pleasures of life – just as 'sometimes foods' and not 'always foods'. Don't put life on hold during your Transform Phase or Balance Phase – you've got to take the stabilizers off in real life.

I hope you enjoy cooking as many of my classic recipes for your family and friends as I do for mine. Just trust your instinct and adapt when needed – especially as far as your children and family are concerned as you know their needs better than anyone.

## ACT AS IF YOU'VE ALREADY GOT IT

Seeing yourself in your new life, five years from now, should feel compelling, exciting and propel you forward. But while you're future-proofing your plan, make sure you don't put your happiness on hold with a 'when I' attitude. Pinning your happiness on a date when you'll 'reach your destination' is to subconsciously say to yourself that in the meantime it's sort of about enduring something miserable. Find your happiness in your habits now. Because if your mind is focusing on what's hard and crappy and all the things you aren't just yet, you're going to find it hard and crappy – and there's so much pleasure to be found now and so much that you already are. The most solid transformations I see are when clients act as if they've already 'got it'.

And while training isn't always hilarious good fun and there are times of the year when you wobble into 50:50, give yourself a break. You're human. Just You Turn as swiftly as you can when you feel grotty – and you'll know when that is. You're meant to have weeks that are looser.

I for one always have to tighten up my habits in January and September, but my mum's Christmas goodies and summer soirées and rosé are truly worth it to me. But I've always got one foot in my habits, even if they're relaxed, so stepping back in seems natural and welcomed. That comes with time but my God, it is so worth it. Maybe it'll take you a few months to find your Balance until you're just living the Lifestyle. You'll never regret how long it took you, just that you didn't find freedom sooner.

Challenge yourself to just start acting as if you've already got the result and you're living your new lifestyle. Think about your new habits as your values, so you're always aligned with them – they're a part of you. It really helped me to think of my lifestyle shift as changing my values. As pretentious as that sounds, do think about it. Keep refining your vision and now start acting like the person that you want to be. Keep acting like the best version of yourself, in this life of balance, enjoying it to the full – and you'll become it. It's up to you to pimp the pleasure up in your New Normal. I can't tell you how important this is. See it as hard work, and it will be. See it as being your choice and being set free, and you will be.

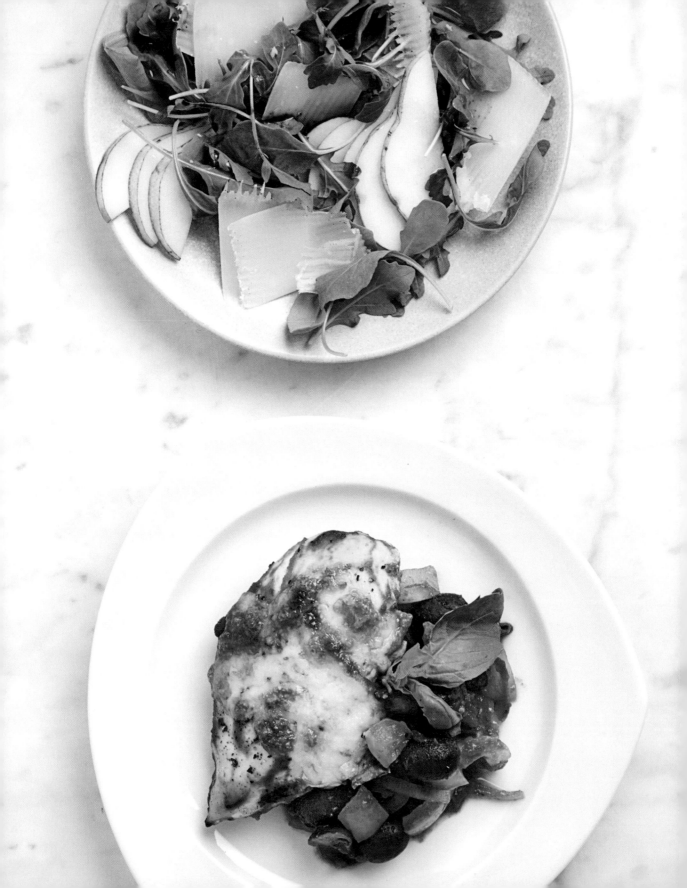

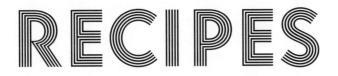

# BREAKFASTS

# ORANGE, HAZELNUT & CINNAMON BIRCHER ⓥ

This citrus purée is worth the effort, so batch it. It's fab spooned on thick Greek yogurt, pancakes or as a smoothie base. Be bold with the cinnamon, these flavours love it.

2 tablespoons jumbo oats
150g (generous ½ cup) low-fat Greek yogurt
4 tablespoons skimmed milk
½ teaspoon vanilla bean paste
½ teaspoon stevia
50g (1¾oz) orange purée
1 teaspoon ground cinnamon
1 tablespoon chopped toasted hazelnuts

### FOR THE ORANGE PURÉE
2 oranges
2 lemons
2 litres (8 cups) water
stevia, to taste

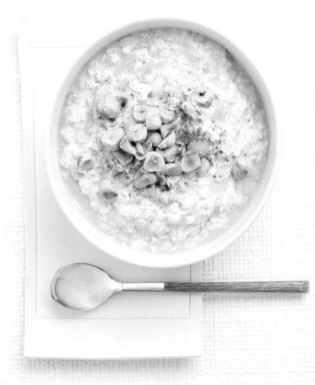

To make the bircher, mix together the oats, yogurt, milk, vanilla and stevia. Cover and leave to soak overnight in the fridge.

For the purée, cut off and discard the ends of the fruit. Now cut the fruit into large wedges. Pop into a saucepan and add the water, making sure the fruit is covered (add more water if not). Bring to the boil, then simmer for 2 hours, topping up with water when necessary.

Drain through a colander and leave the fruit wedges to cool. Whizz in a high-speed blender until lovely and smooth, then stir in the stevia. Chill until ready to serve.

Serve the bircher with 4–5 tablespoons of orange purée marbled through, sprinkled with the cinnamon and chopped hazelnuts.

Store the leftover purée in the fridge for up to 3 days.

# STRAWBERRY & PASSIONFRUIT BIRCHER ⓥ

A firm family favourite. The oatbran is super-high fibre – great for hungrier days. Adjust in the morning with a dash of milk or extra passionfruit for a consistency you love.

SERVES 1

2 tablespoons oatbran
150g (generous ½ cup) low-fat Greek yogurt
4 tablespoons skimmed milk
1 teaspoon vanilla bean paste
125g (⅔ cup) strawberries, sliced
1 teaspoon unsalted pistachios
1 passion fruit

Mix together the oatbran, yogurt, milk and vanilla. Cover and leave to soak overnight in the fridge.

Serve topped with the strawberries, pistachios and seeds and juice scraped from the passion fruit.

# VEGAN CHOCOLATE & RASPBERRY BIRCHER (Vg)

This bircher works beautifully with soya yogurt and feels like pudding for brekkie. Do make extra as you'll want leftovers for snack time.

SERVES 1

2 tablespoons oatbran
200g (¾ cup) unsweetened soya yogurt
½ teaspoon vanilla bean paste
½ teaspoon stevia
4 teaspoons pure cocoa powder
1½ teaspoons cacao nibs
100g (scant 1 cup) fresh raspberries

Mix together the oatbran, soya yogurt, vanilla, stevia, cocoa powder and ½ teaspoon of the cacao nibs. Cover and leave to soak overnight in the fridge.

Roughly crush half the raspberries and fold through the bircher. Serve sprinkled with the remaining raspberries and cacao nibs.

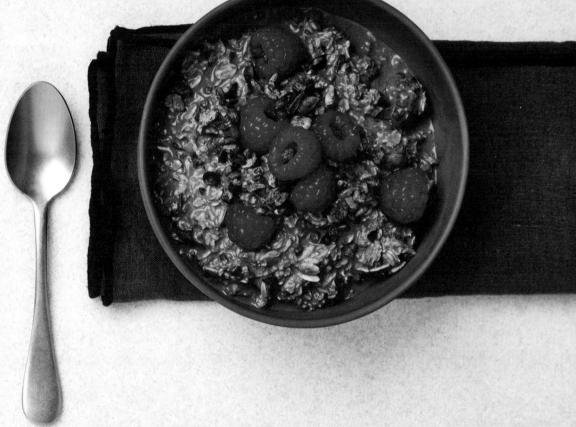

# SPICED BARLEY PORRIDGE (Vg)

Pearl barley has a very satisfying chewy texture and will keep you feeling fuller for longer. The poached pears give this brekkie extra sweetness, and the leftovers can be enjoyed as a snack, whizzed into smoothies or eaten with yogurt.

150g (¾ cup) pearl barley
450ml (scant 2 cups) unsweetened soya milk
250–450ml (1–scant 2 cups) water
¼ teaspoon ground nutmeg
½ teaspoon ground ginger
½ teaspoon ground cinnamon
1 teaspoon stevia
2 tablespoons pumpkin seeds

### FOR THE POACHED PEARS
6 pears, peeled, halved and cored
peeled zest and juice of 1 orange
1 vanilla pod, split in half lengthways
1 cinnamon stick
3 cloves

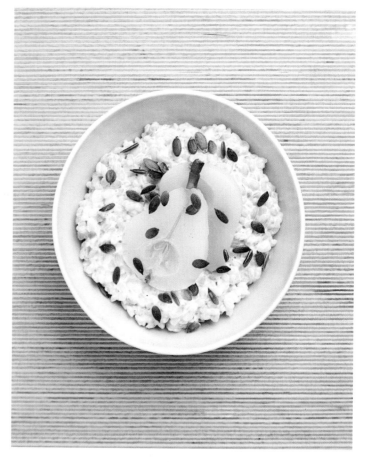

Place the barley in a saucepan with the soya milk, 250ml (1 cup) of the water and the ground spices and cook gently for 30–35 minutes, stirring from time to time, until tender. Add some or all of the extra water if the porridge is looking too dry.

Meanwhile poach the pears. Pop them in a saucepan and add just enough water to cover them. Add the remaining ingredients, bring to the boil and simmer for 10 minutes until they are tender. Leave to cool in the liquid if you have time.

Stir the stevia into the porridge and serve, topping each portion with 2 poached pear halves and a sprinkle of pumpkin seeds.

Store the leftover pears in some of their poaching liquid, covered, in the fridge for up to 4 days.

# QUINOA POWER PORRIDGE Ⓥ

Great for Sunday night prep and works well with soya milk too. Leave to cool, pop in the fridge and scoop out your portion in the morning, heating through with milk or water to your preferred consistency.

small knob of butter
275g (1⅔ cups) quinoa
1 teaspoon stevia
500ml (2 cups) semi-skimmed milk
250ml (1 cup) water
2 apples (skin on), coarsely grated
1 teaspoon vanilla bean paste
1 teaspoon ground cinnamon, plus
a little extra to sprinkle
2 tablespoons low-fat cream cheese
2½ tablespoons chopped toasted hazelnuts

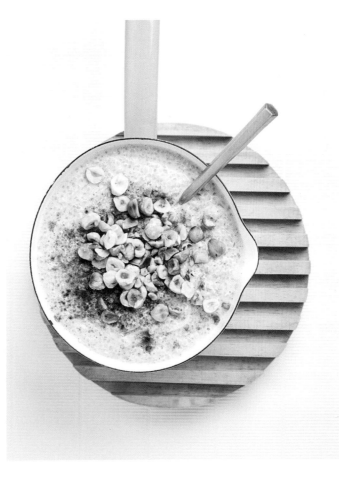

Melt the butter in a large saucepan and gently fry the quinoa until lightly golden – this step adds such a good nutty flavour to the porridge.

Add the stevia, milk and water and simmer for 10 minutes until the quinoa is tender and the porridge has thickened. Add a little more milk or water if it needs a little longer on the hob or is too thick.

Stir in the apples, vanilla, cinnamon and cream cheese and cook for 1 more minute to soften the apples. Serve sprinkled with the hazelnuts and a little more cinnamon.

# COCO'S COCONUT PORRIDGE (Vg)

I love this blend of oats and oatbran with a twist, and it's my youngest's favourite breakfast. Try swapping the rosewater and flowers for grated orange zest and cocoa powder for a chocolate orange twist.

SERVES 2

50g (scant ½ cup) oatbran
50g (½ cup) jumbo oats
450ml (scant 2 cups) unsweetened soya milk
2 tablespoons unsweetened desiccated coconut
½ teaspoon vanilla bean paste
2 drops rosewater
2 tablespoons toasted coconut chips
½ tablespoon dried rose petals

Place the oatbran, jumbo oats, soya milk, desiccated coconut and vanilla in a saucepan over medium heat and bring to a simmer. Cook for 5 minutes until the oats are tender and the porridge has thickened. Add a little more milk or water if it needs a little longer on the hob or is too thick.

Stir in the rosewater and serve sprinkled with coconut chips and rose petals.

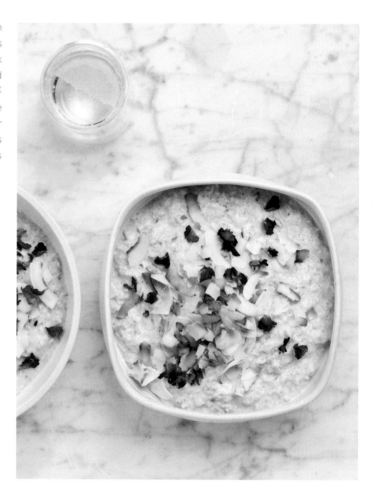

# SWEET BERRY OMELETTE ⓥ

Sounds strange – but the warm oozing berries really work. This protein-packed brekkie makes a great quick supper or lunch too if you feel like something sweet. A hit with my girls.

SERVES 1

2 large eggs
¼ teaspoon stevia
½ teaspoon vanilla bean paste
small knob of unsalted butter
150g (1½ cups) mixed strawberries, blueberries and raspberries

Beat the eggs, stevia and vanilla to combine. Melt the butter in a small nonstick frying pan over medium heat and add the eggs, swirling to coat the pan. Cook for 30 seconds, then sprinkle half the berries over the eggs and cook until the omelette is golden underneath.

Fold up and cook for 20 seconds more. Serve with the remaining berries.

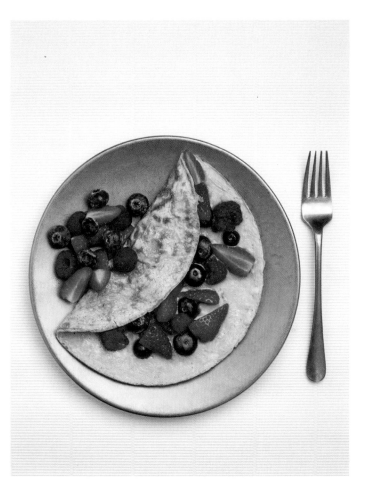

# SOPHIE'S SUPER FLUFFY PANCAKES ⓥ

Nothing beats pancakes at weekends and you won't believe these are so nutritious.
Try with orange zest and the citrus pureé from page 137 – heavenly.

SERVES 4

100g (⅔ cup) wholemeal flour
1½ teaspoons baking powder
1 teaspoon stevia
200g (scant 1 cup) ricotta
finely grated zest and juice of 1 lemon
3 large eggs, separated
1 teaspoon vanilla bean paste
75ml (⅓ cup) skimmed milk
4 teaspoons unsalted butter

FOR THE DRIZZLE
200g (1 cup) strawberries, fresh or frozen
juice of ½ lemon
1 tablespoon mint leaves, chopped

Mix the dry ingredients in a mixing bowl. In a jug, whisk the ricotta, lemon zest and juice, egg yolks, vanilla and milk to combine.

Make a well in the middle of the flour mix, pour in the liquid ingredients and whisk until you get a smooth batter.

Place the egg whites in a separate clean bowl and, using a clean whisk, beat until they hold stiff peaks. Fold the egg whites gently into the batter.

Melt a little of the butter in a large nonstick frying pan over low-medium heat. Add 2 tablespoonfuls of batter for each pancake, cooking 3 or 4 at a time. Flip when the bases are golden and the tops get a few bubbles.

Cook for a couple more minutes until cooked through then keep warm while you cook the remainder. You should end up with 12 in all.

Meanwhile, prepare the drizzle by blending the ingredients together until smooth. Serve the pancakes with the drizzle.

# BANANA PANCAKES
# WITH ALMOND YOGURT (Vg)

This is such a flexible recipe. Experiment and swap in pineapple for banana, peanut butter for almond butter and use Greek yogurt if you want to increase the protein power.

SERVES 4

2 ripe bananas, about 175g (6oz)
150g (1 cup) wholemeal flour
50g (scant ½ cup) oatbran
1 teaspoon baking powder
1 teaspoon stevia
3 tablespoons groundnut oil
1 teaspoon vanilla bean paste
200ml (generous ¾ cup) unsweetened soya milk
200g (scant 2 cups) fresh raspberries

FOR THE ALMOND YOGURT
200g (¾ cup) unsweetened soya yogurt
2 tablespoons almond butter
¼ teaspoon stevia

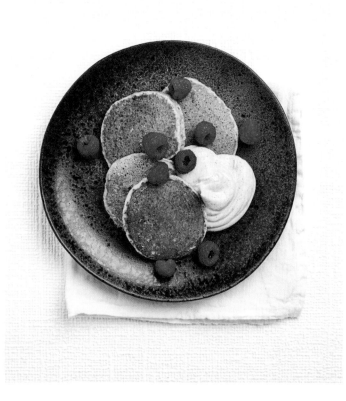

To make the pancake batter, whizz the bananas, flour, oatbran, baking powder, stevia, 2 tablespoons of the oil, the vanilla and milk in a blender until smooth, thick and combined.

Heat a little of the remaining oil in a large nonstick frying pan over low-medium heat. Add 2 tablespoonfuls of the batter to form each pancake, cooking 3 or 4 at a time. Flip the pancakes when the bases are nice and golden and the tops get a few bubbles. Cook for a couple more minutes on the other side until cooked through then keep warm while you cook the remainder. You should end up with 12 in all.

Meanwhile, mix together the ingredients for the almond yogurt.

Serve the pancakes with the almond yogurt and raspberries.

# ALL THE Ps SMOOTHIE ⓥ

Don't tell the kids it has peas in and they'll love it, and always use frozen peas straight
from the freezer. Subtly sweet and protein packed.

150g (generous ½ cup) low-fat Greek yogurt
1 tablespoon oatbran
1 ripe pear (skin on), quartered and cored
25g (scant ¼ cup) frozen peas
50g (½ cup) fresh pineapple chunks
100ml (scant ½ cup) skimmed milk

Blend all the ingredients, ideally using a
high-speed blender, for 1 minute or until
completely smooth.

# STRAWBERRY & AVOCADO SMOOTHIE (v)

Just a fraction of avo in this smoothie adds a wonderful silky texture.

150g (generous ½ cup) low-fat Greek yogurt
125g (⅔ cup) strawberries, fresh or frozen
¼ ripe avocado
1 teaspoon lemon juice
½ teaspoon vanilla bean paste
100ml (scant ½ cup) skimmed milk

Blend all the ingredients, ideally using a high-speed blender, for 1 minute or until completely smooth.

# BEETROOT, APPLE & BLUEBERRY SMOOTHIE (Vg)

A scoop of vegan protein powder works well with the sweetness of the fruit and beetroot. Your skin will love this.

1 tablespoon oatbran
1 scoop vegan protein powder
40g (scant ¼ cup) cooked beetroot
50g (½ cup) blueberries, fresh or frozen
1 apple (skin on), coarsely grated
125ml (½ cup) unsweetened soya milk
¼ teaspoon stevia

Blend all the ingredients, ideally using a high-speed blender, for 1 minute or until completely smooth.

# GREEK AVOCADO TOASTS ⓥ

If I don't have an avocado in the house, I often make these with good-quality hummus spread on the pittas instead. Add an extra squeeze of fresh lemon juice on top to keep it bright and fresh.

SERVES 2

1 ripe avocado, chopped
juice of ½ lemon
2 wholemeal pittas, toasted
100g (scant 1 cup) cherry tomatoes, quartered
¼ cucumber, chopped
25g (¼ cup) pitted Kalamata olives, sliced
25g (scant ¼ cup) feta, crumbled
½ tablespoon chopped dill
sea salt and black pepper

Roughly mash the avocado with the lemon juice and some salt and pepper.

Spread onto the pittas and top with the tomatoes, cucumber and olives. Sprinkle over the feta and dill and serve immediately.

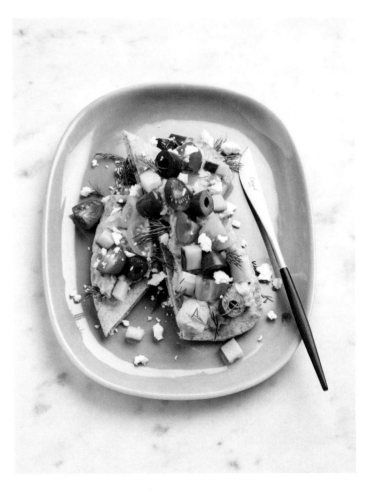

# TEX-MEX BEANS ⓥ

These are dreamy with a poached or fried egg for hungry days. If you can't find chipotle paste, use smoked sweet paprika. Its smoky sweetness is the perfect companion to heaps of fresh herbs and extra lime.

SERVES 4

1 tablespoon olive oil
1 red onion, finely sliced
1 garlic clove, crushed
1 teaspoon chipotle paste
4 tomatoes, roughly chopped
juice of 1 lime
4 soft wholemeal tortillas, warmed
400g (14oz) can black-eyed beans, drained and rinsed
400g (14oz) can kidney beans, drained and rinsed
100g (⅓ cup) low-fat Greek yogurt
¼ teaspoon sweet paprika
handful of coriander leaves, chopped
sea salt and black pepper
lime wedges, to serve

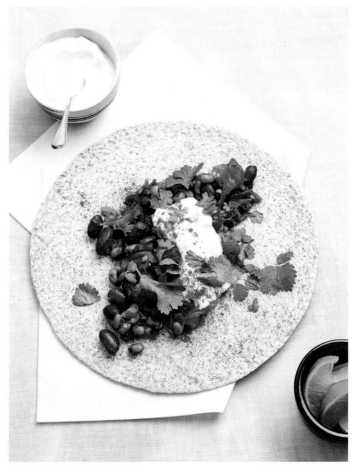

Heat the oil in a saucepan over medium heat and gently sauté the onion and garlic until the onion is translucent.

Stir in the chipotle paste, tomatoes and beans and cook for 5 minutes to soften the tomatoes. Mix in the lime juice and season to taste.

Spoon the beans onto the warm tortillas, top with a dollop of yogurt and sprinkle with paprika and coriander leaves. Serve with lime wedges on the side.

# SALMON, WATERCRESS & CHEDDAR FRITTATA

This works brilliantly with salmon trimmings. I go big on frittatas as they're delicious cold for snacks and packed lunches.

SERVES 4

1 tablespoon olive oil

small knob of unsalted butter

100g (3½oz) watercress, chopped

8 large eggs

2 tablespoons chopped chives

2 spring onions, finely sliced

75g (¾ cup) grated mature Cheddar cheese

125g (4½oz) oak-smoked salmon, sliced

sea salt and black pepper

Preheat the grill to medium.

Heat the oil and butter in a large nonstick frying pan over medium heat and sauté the watercress until just wilted.

Meanwhile, beat the eggs, chives, spring onions and Cheddar really well and season with salt and pepper. Pour into the pan, stirring to mix in the watercress, and cook for 5 minutes until the frittata is set around the edges.

Sprinkle over the smoked salmon and pop under the grill for 5 minutes, keeping an eye on it, until the frittata is set through and lightly golden. Cut into wedges to serve.

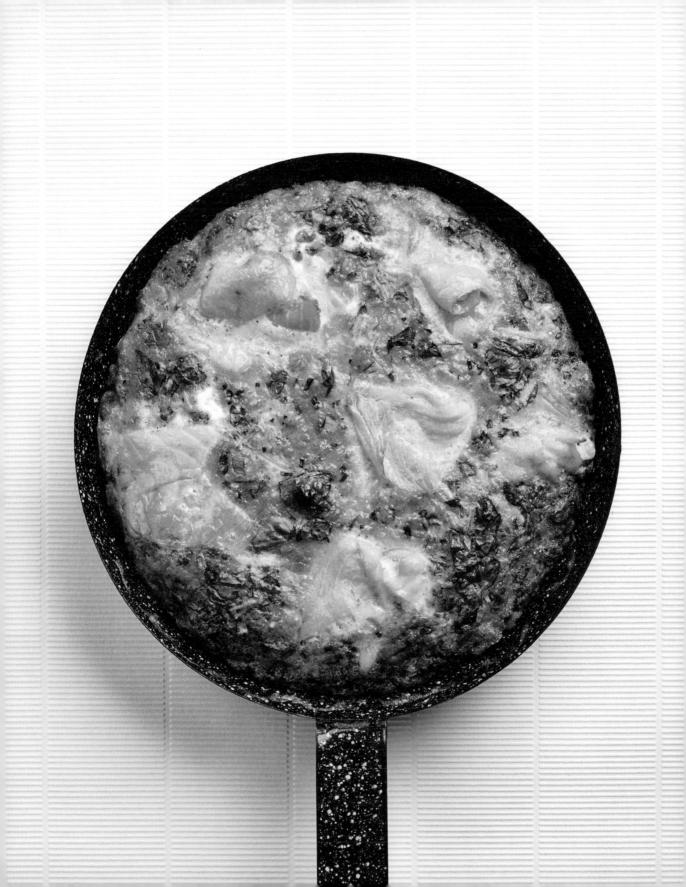

# ASPARAGUS & SMASHED BEAN TARTINES (Vg)

Try this with all sorts of legumes – a great vegan brekkie that is just packed with flavour.

½ teaspoon olive oil
100g (3½oz) asparagus tips
400g (14oz) can cannellini beans, drained and rinsed
1 ripe avocado, chopped
small handful of flat leaf parsley, chopped
zest and juice of ½ lemon
1 tablespoon toasted pine nuts
sea salt and black pepper

### FOR THE TAHINI DRIZZLE
2 tablespoons tahini
1 tablespoon lemon juice
2 tablespoons water

### FOR THE TOASTS
2 slices of good wholemeal bread
½ teaspoon olive oil
1 small garlic clove, peeled

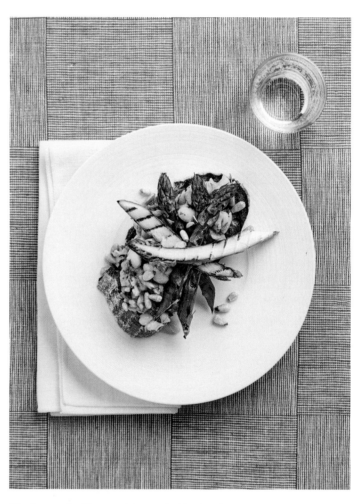

Heat a griddle pan over high heat and brush with the olive oil. Griddle the asparagus until golden and just tender, then set aside and keep warm.

Meanwhile, roughly mash together the cannellini beans, avocado, parsley, lemon zest and juice, and some salt and pepper.

Mix the drizzle ingredients together and season to taste.

To make the toasts, brush the bread with the oil and griddle on both sides until toasted and charred. Rub the garlic clove lightly over the surface of the toast (unless you love garlic, then rub it for longer!).

Pile the mashed bean mixture onto the toasts and top with the asparagus, the tahini drizzle and pine nuts to serve.

# TURKISH BREAKFAST SCRAMBLE ⓥ

This is my take on *menemen*, the just-set egg, tomato and olive oil scramble from Turkey that's so very delicious. It is wonderful topped with a little salty feta.

SERVES 2

1 tablespoon olive oil
small knob of butter
½ red onion, diced
1 orange pepper, cored, deseeded and chopped
1 small garlic clove, crushed
2 plum tomatoes, roughly chopped
4 large eggs
¼ teaspoon dried chilli flakes
small handful of parsley leaves, chopped
2 slices of good wholemeal bread, toasted
25g (scant ¼ cup) feta, crumbled
sea salt and black pepper

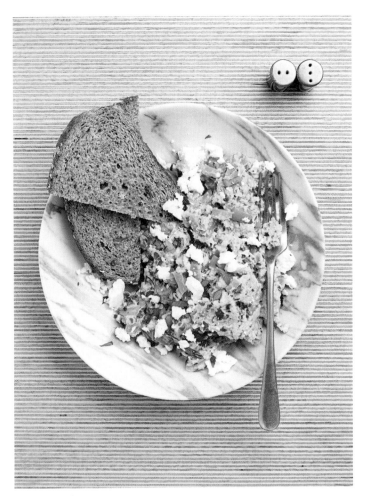

Heat the oil and butter in a nonstick frying pan and gently sauté the onion and pepper for 5 minutes until softened. Add the garlic and tomatoes and keep cooking until the tomatoes have lost most of their moisture. Season to taste.

Meanwhile, beat together the eggs, chilli flakes, parsley and some salt and pepper.

Pour the eggs into the pan and cook, stirring occasionally, until the eggs are just set. Serve immediately on the toast, sprinkled with feta.

# GREEN FRITTERS WITH GOATS' CHEESE & EGG ⓥ

I just adore this for Sunday breakfast with friends. Make sure you really squeeze the liquid out of the courgette. Try it with different cheeses; it also works well with feta and Parmesan.

SERVES 2

1 courgette, coarsely grated

50g (scant ½ cup) broccoli florets, finely chopped

1 spring onion, finely sliced

3 tablespoons wholemeal flour

½ teaspoon baking powder

1 large egg

small handful of parsley leaves, chopped, plus extra to serve

¼ teaspoon sea salt

¼ teaspoon black pepper

1½ tablespoons olive oil

2 large eggs

40g (1½oz) goats' cheese, crumbled

For the fritters, place the veggies, flour, baking powder, egg, parsley, salt and pepper in a large bowl and mix well to make a batter.

Heat 1 tablespoon of the oil in a large nonstick frying pan over medium heat. Add 1 tablespoonful of the batter to form each fritter; you should have enough to make 6. Cook for about 2 minutes, then flip the fritters when the bases are nice and golden. Cook for a couple more minutes on the other side until cooked through. Set aside and keep warm.

Return the pan to the heat and add the remaining oil. Fry the eggs in the oil until done to your liking. Serve the fritters with the fried eggs, sprinkled with the goats' cheese and a little more parsley.

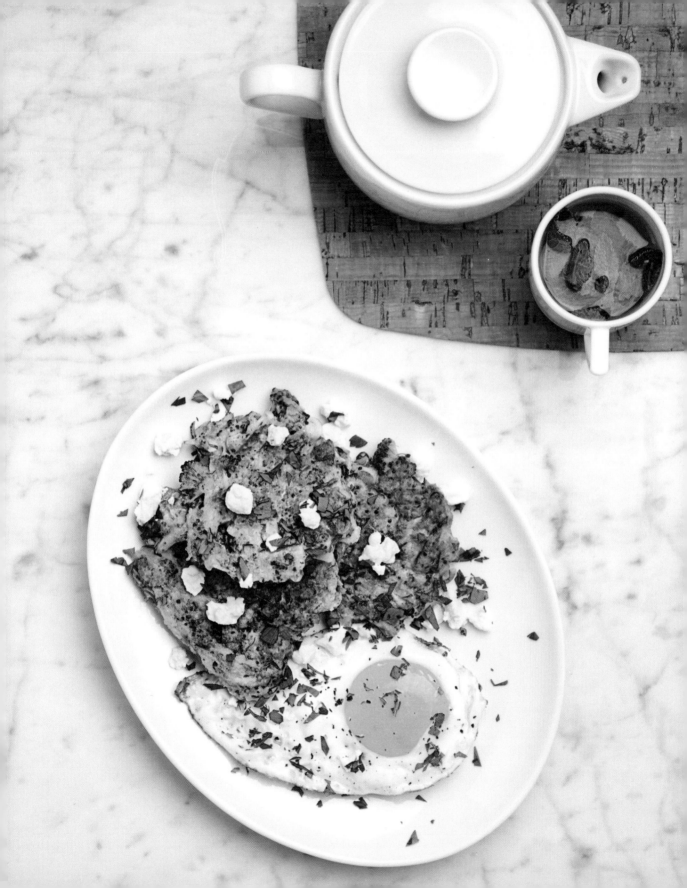

# SNACKS

# CHERRY BERRY SMOOTHIE Ⓥ

My freezer is always full of frozen berries and veg – they're packed with nutrition so stay stocked up.

50g (½ cup) fresh or frozen raspberries
100g (1 cup) frozen cherries
100g (⅓ cup) low-fat Greek yogurt
1 tablespoon oatbran
100ml (scant ½ cup) skimmed milk

Blend all the ingredients, ideally using a high-speed blender, for 1 minute or until completely smooth.

SERVES 1

# PEANUT BUTTER & JELLY SMOOTHIE Ⓥg

The combination of sugar-free peanut butter with ripe or frozen strawberries works an American dream. Soya yogurt is lower in protein than Greek so add a little vanilla vegan protein powder to turn this into a higher protein meal.

1 tablespoon sugar-free peanut butter

4 teaspoons oatbran

100ml (scant ½ cup) unsweetened almond or soya milk

75g (generous ¼ cup) plain soya yogurt

½ teaspoon vanilla bean paste

100g (½ cup) strawberries

Blend the peanut butter, 3 teaspoons oatbran, milk, yogurt and vanilla, ideally using a high-speed blender, for 1 minute or until completely smooth. Pour into a glass.

Give the blender a quick rinse, then whizz the strawberries and remaining oatbran to a purée. Pour on top of the smoothie to form a separate layer.

# ROASTED AUBERGINE & RICOTTA DIP ⓥ

I love dips for their ease – pack into a little box with oatcakes, a toasted mini wholemeal pitta or some chopped veggies for a snack on the go. Or spread some on a slice of good wholemeal toast, top with a soft-boiled egg and you have a stellar breakfast. This one keeps well in the fridge too. One portion is 2 tablespoons with 2 oatcakes.

1 aubergine, halved lengthways
2 tablespoons olive oil
½ teaspoon ground sumac
75g (2¾oz) ricotta
75g (2¾oz) low-fat Greek yogurt
finely grated zest and juice of ½ lemon
¼ teaspoon sea salt
¼ teaspoon black pepper
small handful of parsley leaves, finely chopped
25g (¼ cup) walnut pieces
oatcakes, pittas or crudités, to serve

Preheat the oven to 200°C/400°F/Gas Mark 6.

Make deep cuts in a criss-cross pattern into the cut sides of the aubergine halves to speed up cooking, then brush with a little of the oil. Place on a baking sheet, cut sides up, sprinkle over the sumac and cook in the oven for 40 minutes or until really tender.

Use a spoon to scoop the aubergine flesh into a blender and discard the skins. Add the remaining oil to the blender with the ricotta, yogurt, lemon zest and juice, salt, pepper and most of the parsley and walnuts. Whizz until smooth. Taste for seasoning, adding more if you like.

Transfer to a bowl, sprinkle over the remaining parsley and nuts and serve with oatcakes, pittas or crudités. Store the leftover dip, covered, in the fridge for up to 4 days.

# AVOCADO & ARTICHOKE DIP Ⓥ

This mild and creamy dip is wonderful and needs to be eaten on the day it's made. Use plenty of lime and cover in clingfilm to keep the vibrant green colour. Spread on a couple of oatcakes or crispbread or, if you're in a lighter mood, serve with crunchy crudités.

MAKES 2 PORTIONS

½ ripe avocado, chopped
35g (1¼oz) chargrilled artichokes in oil, drained
50g (scant ¼ cup) low-fat Greek yogurt
10g (¼oz) feta
½ tablespoon chopped chives
squeeze of lemon juice
sea salt and black pepper
oatcakes or crudités, to serve

Place all the ingredients in a blender and whizz until smooth. Taste for seasoning, adding more salt, pepper or lemon juice if you like.

Transfer to a bowl and serve with oatcakes or crudités.

# ROASTED
# EDAMAME BEANS (Vg)

These roasted beans are full of protein and really portable. I use frozen which seem to cook better. Try with chilli flakes instead of paprika for a hotter hit. Make sure you cool them thoroughly before storing in an airtight container (refresh them for a few minutes in a dry, hot frying pan on the day you plan to eat them).

600g (4 cups) frozen shelled edamame beans
½ teaspoon garlic granules
½ teaspoon sea salt
½ teaspoon black pepper
1 teaspoon smoked sweet paprika

Preheat the oven to 180°C/350°F/Gas Mark 4.

Place all the ingredients in a large bowl, mix well and spread out in a single layer on a baking tray lined with baking paper. Bake for 45 minutes, turning occasionally, until golden and almost crispy – take them out too soon and they can go soggy. Sometimes I even give mine a quick blast under the grill for extra crispiness.

Allow to cool completely on the tray. Store in an airtight container for up to 4 days.

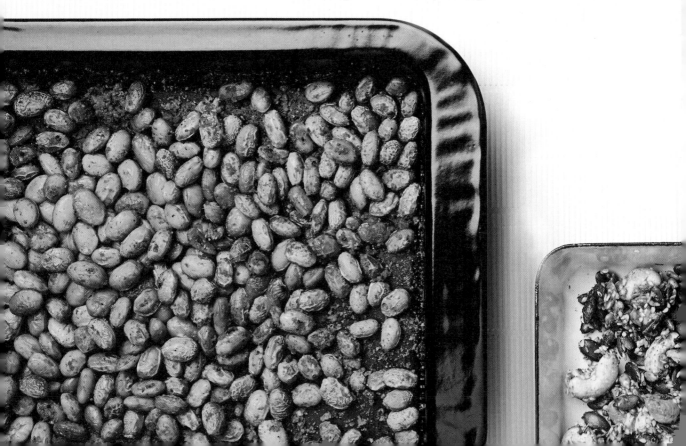

# CASHEWS & SEEDS ⓥ

These nuts are very moreish. One portion is 2 heaped tablespoons so portion up before you get too carried away, and eat them with a portion of low GI fruit. They stay fantastically crunchy in a jar for well over a week.

2 teaspoons finely chopped rosemary
1 small egg white
¼ teaspoon cayenne pepper
½ teaspoon ground cumin
100g (1 cup) unsalted cashews
2 tablespoons pumpkin seeds
2 tablespoons sunflower seeds
1 tablespoon sesame seeds
sea salt and black pepper

Preheat the oven to 180°C/350°F/Gas Mark 4.

Place the rosemary, egg white and spices in a bowl and mix well, breaking up the egg white. Season with salt and pepper.

Stir in the cashews and seeds and mix until everything is nicely coated. Scrape onto a baking tray lined with baking paper and spread out in an even layer.

Bake for about 15 minutes until golden, breaking up the mixture into small clusters after about 10 minutes.

Leave to cool completely. You might need to break up the clusters a little more once the mixture is cool. Store in an airtight container for up to 2 weeks.

# SAVOURY GRANOLA ⓥ

A handful (2 heaped tablespoons) of savoury granola and a piece of fruit makes a fast snack. I also love this sprinkled on a soup to give an amazing crunch. Or serve a spoonful over your poached eggs on toast for a very trendy start to the day.

50g (scant ½ cup) pumpkin seeds
100g (1 cup) jumbo oats
1 tablespoon sesame seeds
50g (½ cup) pecans
1 teaspoon fennel seeds
¼ teaspoon dried chilli flakes
1 tablespoon reduced-sodium soy sauce
1 tablespoon olive oil
⅛ teaspoon sea salt
1 egg white

Preheat the oven to 180°C/350°F/Gas Mark 4.

Place all the ingredients in a large bowl, mix well and spread on a small baking tray lined with baking paper – not too thinly or the mixture may burn. Bake for 15–20 minutes, stirring occasionally, until toasted and golden.

Allow to cool completely on the tray. Store in an airtight container for up to a week.

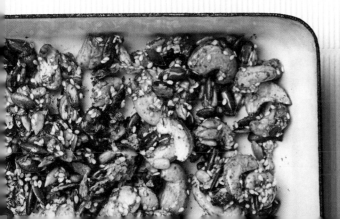

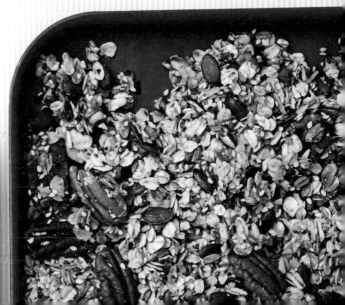

# RUBY RED TARTINE ⓥ

SERVES 1

So simple to make and a way to make cottage cheese – a great but boring protein – sexy. Works beautifully with my Vitality Sauce (see *Lean for Life: The Cookbook*, page 54) and Summer Berry Compote (see *The Louise Parker Method: Lean for Life*, page 80).

2 tablespoons cottage cheese
1½ tablespoons low-fat cream cheese
¼ teaspoon stevia
¼ teaspoon vanilla bean paste
½ teaspoon finely grated orange zest
1 small slice of good wholemeal bread, toasted
2–3 strawberries, sliced
½ tablespoon pomegranate seeds

Place the cottage cheese, cream cheese, stevia, vanilla and orange zest in a bowl and mix well.

Spread on the toast and top with the strawberries and pomegranate seeds.

# MONKEY TOAST ⓥ

SERVES 1

My girls just love Monkey Toast, I think largely due to the name. Try it with almond or hazelnut butter and ring the changes with different nuts and seeds. Great with a cup of tea when you need a comforting afternoon take-out-treat snack.

1½ tablespoons low-fat Greek yogurt
1 tablespoon sugar-free crunchy peanut butter
⅛ teaspoon stevia
1 small slice of good wholemeal bread, toasted
¼ banana, thinly sliced
1 teaspoon toasted flaked almonds

Place the yogurt, peanut butter and stevia in a bowl and mix well.

Spread on the toast and top with the banana slices and almonds.

# CINNAMON CHIPS
# WITH CHOCOLATE DIP ⓥ

These chips never last long in our house – but if they did, they could be kept in an airtight box for well over a week, so it makes sense to make a big batch. I also make a savoury version, sprinkling them with smoked paprika – perfect to serve with the dips on pages 158–9. I sometimes add some orange zest to this lovely chocolate dip. In the Lifestyle Phase or for a kids' snack, I use full-fat Greek yogurt. Leftovers are great for a smoothie base, so batch away.

2 wholemeal tortillas
1 teaspoon vegetable oil
½ teaspoon ground cinnamon
½ teaspoon stevia

FOR THE DIP
200g (¾ cup) low-fat Greek yogurt
1 teaspoon vanilla bean paste
1 tablespoon pure cocoa powder, sifted
1 teaspoon stevia
½ tablespoon chopped roasted hazelnuts

Preheat the oven to 180°C/350°F/Gas Mark 4.

Brush the tortillas with the oil – I find rubbing them together with a little oil between them makes for a quick covering! Mix together the cinnamon and stevia and sprinkle on the tortillas.

Cut into triangles, arrange in a single layer on a baking tray and bake for 10–15 minutes, turning midway through, until crisp. Watch them carefully as they go from nice and golden to burned quite quickly. Allow to cool completely.

For the dip, mix all the ingredients, except the hazelnuts, in a bowl until well combined. Sprinkle the hazelnuts over the top. That's it.

The chips can be stored in an airtight container for up to 10 days. Store the dip, covered, in the fridge for up to 3 days. Stir before serving to avoid separation.

# GRIDDLED NECTARINE WITH
# BUFFALO MOZZARELLA ⓥ

Griddling the nectarine makes it even juicier and the charring adds another
level of flavour, but if you're in a rush you can, of course, leave this step out.
This combination also makes a lovely summer starter.

SERVES 1

1 nectarine, halved and stoned
½ teaspoon olive oil
50g (1¾oz) buffalo mozzarella, torn into
pieces
pinch of chilli flakes
a few mint leaves

Brush the cut sides of the nectarine with the
olive oil.

Heat a griddle pan over a high heat then griddle
the nectarine halves until charred and stripy.

Serve with the mozzarella, sprinkled with chilli
flakes and mint leaves.

# LITTLE PIZZA MARGHERITAS (v)

A speedy snack which definitely satisfies any fast-food cravings! You can try different toppings to replicate your favourite pizza flavours. Sliced black olives are another great (and easy) addition.

MAKES 4 PORTIONS

4 mini wholemeal pittas, or 2 normal pittas, halved and toasted

1¼ tablespoons tomato purée

½ teaspoon dried oregano

75g (2¾oz) mozzarella, chopped

a few small basil leaves

Preheat the grill to high.

Spread the tomato purée on top of the toasted pittas, then sprinkle over the oregano and mozzarella.

Grill until golden and bubbling. Top with the basil and enjoy.

# MAINS

# HERBY CHICKEN, PEACH & FETA SALAD

SERVES 2

I love this sweet and salty combination. Simply one of my favourite summer salads, this also works well with barbecued chicken, nectarines or fresh figs. Go heavy on the herbs for extra zing.

2 ripe peaches, halved and stoned
½ tablespoon olive oil
200g (7oz) cooked chicken, shredded
small handful of mint leaves, chopped
small handful of basil leaves, chopped
2 tablespoons chopped chives
75g (2¾oz) pea shoots
75g (2¾oz) feta, crumbled
50g (½ cup) walnuts, chopped

**FOR THE DRESSING**
1 teaspoon wholegrain mustard
1½ tablespoons extra virgin olive oil
finely grated zest of 1 lime
juice of ½ lime

Heat a griddle pan over high heat. Brush the peaches with the oil and griddle, cut side down, until lovely and charred.

Meanwhile, mix the dressing ingredients together in a large bowl and toss in the chicken, herbs and pea shoots.

Serve the chicken mixture topped with the luscious griddled peaches, the feta and walnuts.

# LEAN GREEN SALAD

This very green salad takes moments to make. Soya beans give an extra dose of protein and are always on hand in the freezer. The orange dressing is light and gives a little taste of sweetness.

SERVES 2

125g (1 cup) frozen soya beans
150g (5½oz) cooked chicken, chopped
½ cucumber, chopped
1 ripe avocado, chopped
1 Romaine lettuce, thickly sliced
125g (scant 1 cup) green beans, cooked and cooled
2 tablespoons pumpkin seeds

FOR THE DRESSING
finely grated zest and juice of 1 orange
2 tablespoons chopped chives
½ tablespoon wholegrain mustard
1 tablespoon extra virgin olive oil
sea salt and black pepper

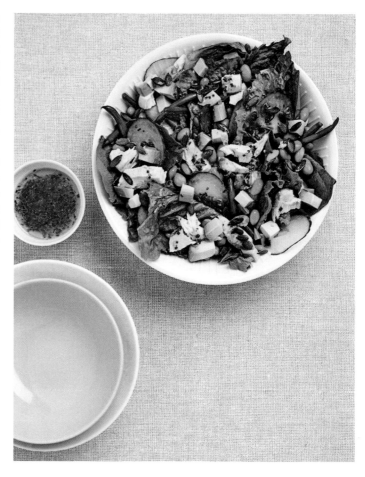

Defrost the soya beans in a bowl of just-boiled water. Drain well. Tip into a salad bowl and add the remaining salad ingredients, except for the pumpkin seeds.

Mix the dressing ingredients and pour into the salad bowl. Toss to dress the salad, sprinkle over the pumpkin seeds and you're ready.

# FRUITY MACKEREL SALAD

Mackerel is a great fridge standby that weirdly works wonderfully with fruit. Do try it and use the best orange that you can find to really make this salad zing.

SERVES 2

150g (5½oz) smoked mackerel fillets, flaked
200g (1 cup) cooked beetroot, chopped
100g (3½oz) watercress
1 orange, cut into segments
2 tablespoons pumpkin seeds
2 tablespoons chopped chives

### FOR THE DRESSING
2 tablespoons extra virgin olive oil
finely grated zest and juice of 1 lemon
1 teaspoon Dijon mustard
sea salt and black pepper

Place all the dressing ingredients in a large bowl, mix well and season to taste. Mix through the mackerel, beetroot, watercress and orange segments. Sprinkle over the pumpkin seeds and chives and it's ready to serve.

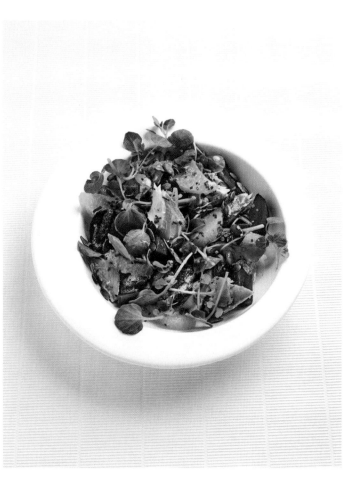

SERVES 4

# SOPHIE'S SUMMER GAZPACHO (Vg)

My eldest daughter's favourite summer soup, and simple enough for her to make. An authentic gazpacho is made with bread, giving it that unique texture, but I've swapped the bread for butterbeans, which add creaminess and protein. This is a great recipe for making in advance because it's at its best when it's had a day to rest in the fridge.

1 cucumber, peeled and chopped

1 red pepper, cored, deseeded and chopped

1 green pepper, cored, deseeded and chopped

800g (1lb 12oz) very ripe plum tomatoes, chopped

3 spring onions, chopped

2 garlic cloves, chopped

1 tablespoon red wine vinegar

2 tablespoons extra virgin olive oil, plus extra to serve

½ teaspoon paprika

½ teaspoon sea salt

½ teaspoon black pepper

400g (14oz) can butterbeans, drained and rinsed

Put all the ingredients into a high-speed blender and give them a really good whizz until extra smooth. Taste and check whether the consistency and seasoning are right for you; if not add a little water or more salt and pepper.

Pop in the fridge until really cold – this also gives the flavours time to mingle. Serve with a simple swirl of olive oil.

# GREEK SALAD FRITTATA ⓥ

I love frittatas as they are so endlessly adaptable. You really can raid your fridge and get a great result. Try baking in a square baking tin to cut into little squares for snacks and lunchboxes

SERVES 4

1 tablespoon olive oil
small knob of unsalted butter
1 red onion, finely sliced
1 large courgette, coarsely grated
50g (½ cup) pitted Kalamata olives
200g (1½ cups) cherry tomatoes
8 large eggs
handful of parsley leaves, chopped
150g (5½oz) feta, crumbled or chopped
sea salt and black pepper

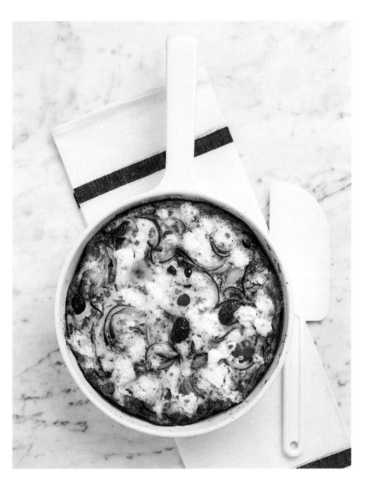

Preheat the grill to medium.

Heat the oil and butter in a large nonstick frying pan over medium heat and fry the onion and courgette until lightly cooked. Stir in the olives and tomatoes and fry gently until the tomatoes become gooey and the liquid has cooked off.

Meanwhile, beat the eggs and parsley really well and season with salt and pepper. Pour into the pan, stirring to mix in the veg, and cook for 5 minutes until the frittata is set around the edges.

Sprinkle over the feta and pop under the grill for 5 minutes, keeping an eye on it, until the frittata is set through and lightly golden. Serve in wedges.

# SHAVED FENNEL & PRAWN SALAD

I love this refreshing salad on a hot day. If you are feeling fancy, you can pan-fry some scallops to serve with the salad instead of adding the prawns. Fennel bulbs can vary quite considerably in size, so if you have a little one use it all.

SERVES 2

½ fennel bulb
1 Granny Smith apple
150g (5½oz) cooked, peeled and deveined king prawns
6 radishes, finely sliced
2 handfuls of lambs' lettuce
1 ripe avocado, sliced

FOR THE DRESSING
finely grated zest and juice of 1 lemon
½ tablespoon red wine vinegar
1 teaspoon Dijon mustard
2 tablespoons chopped dill
2 tablespoons rapeseed oil
sea salt and black pepper

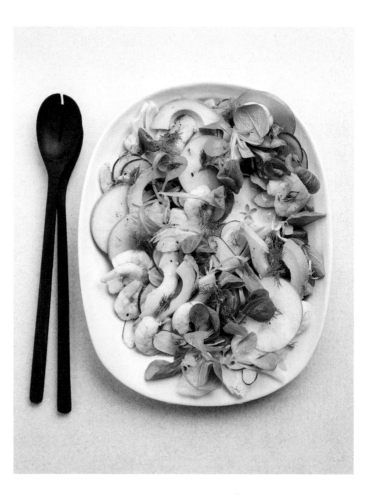

Place all the dressing ingredients in a large bowl, mix well and season to taste.

Use a mandolin to finely slice the fennel straight into the dressing bowl, coating it in the dressing to stop it going brown.

Halve and core the apple and slice on the mandolin in the same way. Add the prawns, radishes and lambs' lettuce to the bowl and toss all the salad ingredients together. Serve with the sliced avocado.

# CRUNCHY SHREDDED CHICKEN SALAD

I usually make my salad dressings in the bottom of a salad bowl, then I can easily toss all the other ingredients straight into it and make sure they are nicely coated. Saves on the washing up too. This works so well with leftover roast meats.

SERVES 2

200g (7oz) cooked chicken, shredded
¼ small red cabbage, cored and finely shredded

⅓ cucumber, chopped
2 carrots, cut into matchsticks or spiralized
50g (⅔ cup) baby spinach
2 tablespoons pumpkin seeds

### FOR THE DRESSING
½ tablespoon white wine vinegar
1 tablespoon extra virgin olive oil
½ tablespoon Dijon mustard
2 tablespoons tahini
finely grated zest and juice of 1 lemon
1 tablespoon water
sea salt and black pepper

Mix the dressing ingredients together in a large bowl. Toss through all the salad ingredients, except the pumpkin seeds.

Serve in bowls with the seeds scattered over the top.

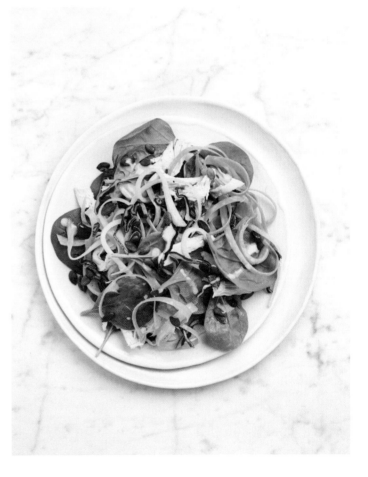

# COCO'S CORONATION

This salad is so speedy and the mild curry is a great way to introduce spice to little people. I often make a batch of this for work and midweek suppers for Paul and I, then pop the mixture into wholemeal wraps for the girls after school. Great for batching.

SERVES 2

100g (⅓ cup) low-fat Greek yogurt
1 ripe peach, peeled, stoned and chopped
1 tablespoon mild curry paste
¼ teaspoon sea salt
150g (5½oz) cooked chicken, cut into strips
1 apple, cored and chopped
2 celery sticks, chopped
50g (½ cup) walnuts, chopped
2 spring onions, finely sliced
handful of parsley leaves, chopped
200g (1¼ cups) green beans, cooked and cooled
1 Baby Gem lettuce, thickly sliced

Whizz the yogurt, peach, curry paste and salt in a blender until smooth.

Empty into a large bowl and mix in the chicken, apple, celery, walnuts, spring onions and parsley.

Serve the chicken mixture on a bed of beans and lettuce.

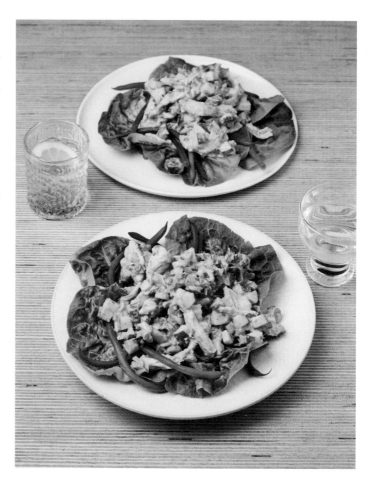

# CRUNCHY CRAB SALAD

I adore crab and this always cheers me up – the richness works so well with the crunchy fresh veg. If I have time I'll toast the cashew nuts too. If you prefer your beansprouts cooked, fry them in a hot pan with a teaspoon of oil for 2 minutes.

1 Little Gem lettuce, shredded

½ cucumber, chopped

2 carrots, coarsely grated

100g (1 cup) beansprouts

150g (5½oz) white and brown crab meat, or just white if you prefer

1 tablespoon white or black sesame seeds

1 tablespoon chopped chives

25g (⅓ cup) unsalted cashew nuts, chopped

## FOR THE DRESSING

½ tablespoon groundnut oil

½ tablespoon toasted sesame oil

½ green chilli, finely chopped

1 tablespoon reduced-sodium soy sauce

Place all the dressing ingredients in a large bowl and mix well. Add all the salad ingredients, toss well to combine and taste, adding a little more soy sauce if you like. So simple, so tasty!

# TUNA TOSSED SALAD

A super-speedy salad which is great for packing into a lunchbox as none of the ingredients will wilt. Griddled tuna steaks cut into cubes take this up a notch.

2 celery sticks, chopped
1 red pepper, cored, deseeded and chopped
⅓ cucumber, quartered lengthways and thickly sliced
100g (scant 1 cup) cherry tomatoes, halved
200g (7oz) can tuna steak in brine or spring water, drained
400g (14oz) can butterbeans, drained and rinsed
2 tablespoons sunflower seeds

### FOR THE DRESSING
1 teaspoon thyme leaves
1 tablespoon red wine vinegar
1 shallot, finely chopped
2 tablespoons extra virgin olive oil
sea salt and black pepper

Mix the dressing ingredients together in a large bowl and add all the salad ingredients. Toss to coat everything in the dressing and serve.

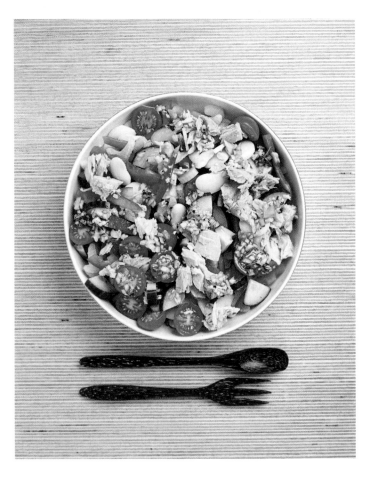

# THE GREAT VEG FRITTATA ⓥ

Use the best eggs that you can and play around with different veggies and cheeses.
A really simple midweek supper and also fab eaten cold the next day.

SERVES 4

1 tablespoon olive oil
small knob of unsalted butter
1 parsnip, coarsely grated
2 carrots, coarsely grated
1 large courgette, coarsely grated
8 large eggs
3 tablespoons chopped chives
125g (1¼ cups) grated mature
Cheddar cheese
sea salt and black pepper

Preheat the grill to medium.

Heat the oil and butter in a large nonstick
frying pan over medium heat and fry the
veggies until lightly cooked.

Meanwhile, beat the eggs, chives and cheese
really well and season with salt and pepper.
Pour into the pan, stirring to mix in the veg,
and cook for 5 minutes until the frittata is set
around the edges.

Pop under the grill for 5 minutes, keeping an
eye on it, until the frittata is set through and
lightly golden. Serve in wedges.

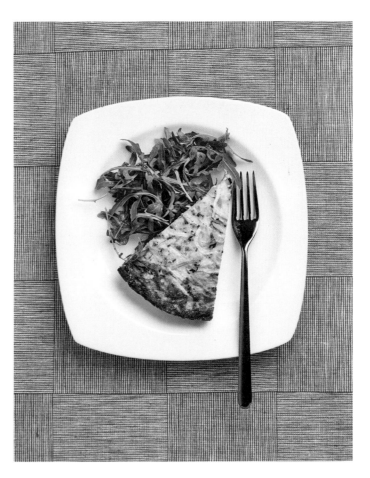

# VIETNAMESE-STYLE PORK 'NOODLE' SALAD

This salad has such a great flavour and crunch. You could use skinless chicken thighs instead of the pork if you prefer. And if you don't have a spiralizer, you can of course cut the carrots and courgettes into matchsticks. There's a really good dose of protein in this one so it's great for hungrier days.

1 teaspoon groundnut oil

225g (8oz) pork loin medallions or chops (visible fat trimmed), sliced

125g (1 cup) frozen soya beans, cooked

1 red pepper, cored, deseeded and thinly sliced

1 yellow pepper, cored, deseeded and thinly sliced

2 carrots, spiralized into 'noodles'

1 courgette, spiralized into 'noodles'

leaves from 1 bunch of coriander, chopped

### FOR THE DRESSING

1 tablespoon peeled and grated fresh root ginger

2 tablespoons reduced-sodium soy sauce

finely grated zest and juice of 1 lime

1 teaspoon sesame seeds

1 teaspoon toasted sesame oil

1 tablespoon crunchy peanut butter

½ red chilli, finely chopped

2 tablespoons water

Mix all the dressing ingredients together in a large bowl and have a taste, adding a little more soy sauce if you like. The dressing is what makes this salad, so take a little time tasting it to see if it's how you want it.

Next heat the oil in a nonstick frying pan over medium-high heat, add the pork and cook until it is nicely caramelized and cooked through. Transfer to the dressing bowl and toss to let the pork start soaking up the flavours.

Gently mix through all the vegetables, sprinkle over the coriander and serve.

# SAMUI SALMON BURGERS

These work brilliantly with a little Indian curry paste too, and with ground pork or chicken. Wonderful for barbecues. I batch and freeze them in clingfilm.

SERVES 4

600g (1lb 5oz) skinless salmon fillets
2 teaspoons Thai green curry paste
2 tablespoons peeled and grated fresh root ginger
large handful of fresh coriander, roughly chopped
finely grated zest of 1 lime
1 teaspoon groundnut oil
sea salt and black pepper

### FOR THE SALAD
1 cucumber
150g (2 cups) sugar snap peas, shredded
2 spring onions, shredded
1 teaspoon sesame oil
juice of ½ lime
1 tablespoon black and white sesame seeds
50g (½ cup) cashew nuts, roasted and chopped
handful of flat leaf parsley leaves, finely chopped

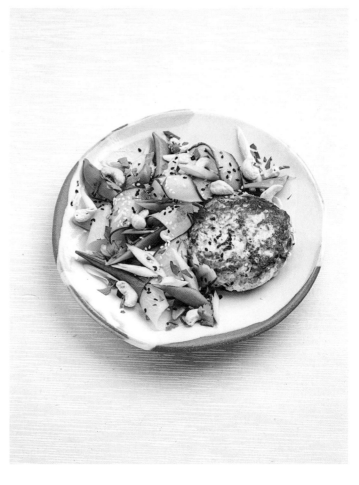

Put the salmon into a food processor with the curry paste, ginger, coriander and lime zest, season to taste and whizz until finely chopped and coming together. Shape into 4 flattened patties, cover and chill for 10 minutes to firm up.

Meanwhile, use a vegetable peeler to peel the cucumber into ribbons, discarding the inner seedy core. Put into a salad bowl with the remaining salad ingredients and toss to coat. Set aside.

Heat the oil in a large nonstick frying pan and fry the salmon burgers for 10 minutes, turning once, until cooked through. Serve the burgers with the salad.

# PIZZA CHICKEN TRAYBAKE

My daughters love this recipe – it tastes so much like pizza! It's light on the washing up because you don't have to do any browning of meat or onions before it goes in the oven, and it freezes really well too – the dream weeknight supper.

SERVES 4

2 x 400g (14oz) cans chopped tomatoes
2 tablespoons tomato purée
1 teaspoon dried oregano
small handful of basil leaves
2 yellow peppers, cored, deseeded and cut into chunks
1 red onion, finely sliced
150g (2 cups) mushrooms, sliced
50g (½ cup) pitted black olives
4 skinless chicken breasts, about 150g (5½oz) each
100g (3½oz) mozzarella, chopped
sea salt and black pepper

### FOR THE SALAD
2 tablespoons extra virgin olive oil
1 tablespoon aged balsamic vinegar
70g (2½oz) rocket
1 pear (skin on) cored and finely sliced
25g (¼ cup) finely grated pecorino or Parmesan

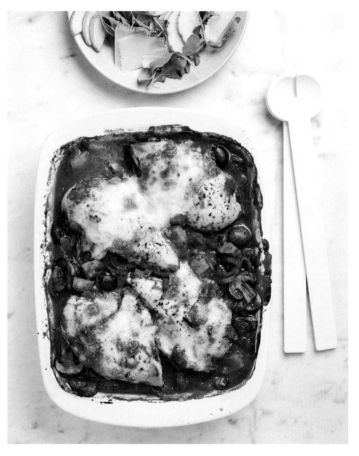

Preheat the oven to 200°C/400°F/Gas Mark 6.

Place all the ingredients, except for the chicken and cheese, in a large ovenproof dish and bake for 15 minutes, giving the mixture an occasional stir.

Remove from the oven and add the chicken, spooning over the sauce to cover it. Return to the oven for 45 minutes until the chicken is cooked through, sprinkling over the cheese for the final 10 minutes.

To make the salad, mix the olive oil and balsamic vinegar in a large bowl, add the rocket, pear and pecorino or Parmesan and gently toss.

Serve the salad with the chicken.

# LOVELY LENTIL BAKE (v)

This makes a spicy chilli bake – add less chilli if you prefer, or remove the seeds for a milder taste. You can make the lentil mixture ahead of time, and chill or freeze it until ready to serve. Then defrost if necessary, sprinkle with the cheese and bake until piping hot.

SERVES 4

1 tablespoon olive oil

1 large red onion, chopped

2 garlic cloves, finely chopped

2 celery sticks, chopped

2 carrots, coarsely grated

1 large courgette, coarsely grated

3 tablespoons tomato purée

2 x 400g (14oz) cans green lentils, drained and rinsed

400g (14oz) can chopped tomatoes

500ml (2 cups) good vegetable stock

2 red chillies, finely chopped

1 teaspoon hot smoked paprika

1 teaspoon dried oregano

½ teaspoon sea salt

½ teaspoon black pepper

50g (½ cup) grated mature Cheddar cheese

### FOR THE SALSA

2 ripe avocados, chopped

finely grated zest and juice of 1 lime

leaves from 1 bunch of coriander, chopped

2 spring onions, sliced

4 tomatoes, roughly chopped

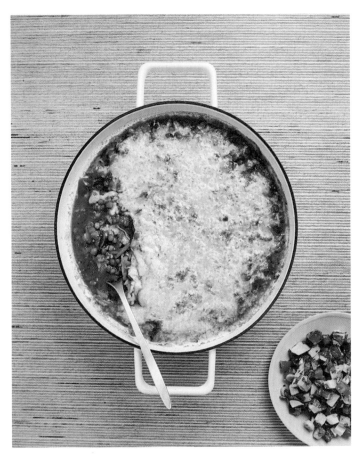

Preheat the oven to 180°C/350°F/Gas Mark 4.

Heat the oil in a large frying pan and sweat the onion, garlic and celery until translucent, about 10 minutes. Stir in all the remaining ingredients apart from the Cheddar and simmer for 15 minutes until thick and lovely. Taste and adjust the seasoning as you like.

When ready to serve, transfer the mixture to an ovenproof casserole dish and sprinkle over the Cheddar. Bake for 20 minutes until the mixture is piping hot and the cheese is golden and bubbling.

Meanwhile, make the salsa by mixing together all the ingredients and seasoning to taste. Serve with the chilli.

# SPICED CARROT & RED LENTIL SOUP (Vg)

I also love to top this soup with crumbled goats' cheese when I have some in the fridge. This is another soup that lends itself to batch-cooking and freezing in portions for an instant meal.

SERVES 4

1 teaspoon rapeseed oil, plus extra to drizzle
1 onion, finely chopped
3 large carrots, finely chopped
1 teaspoon ground ginger
1 teaspoon paprika
½ teaspoon ground turmeric
300g (1½ cups) dried red lentils, rinsed in cold water
800ml (3¼ cups) good vegetable stock
2 tablespoons pumpkin seeds
sea salt and black pepper

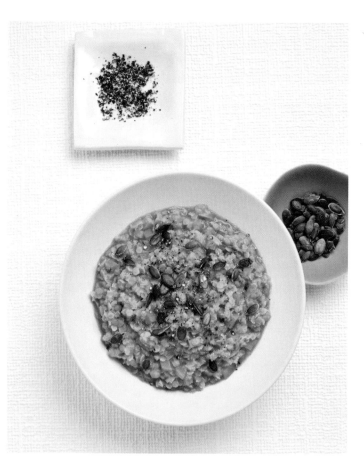

Heat the oil in a large saucepan over medium heat and gently sauté the onion and carrots until the onions are translucent. Now add the spices and lentils and fry until the spices are fragrant and toasted.

Stir in the stock and simmer gently for 20 minutes until the lentils are tender. I like this soup as it is, but feel free to blend it if you prefer a smooth texture.

Season to taste and serve sprinkled with the pumpkin seeds and a little drizzle of oil.

# MILLY'S MIXED BEAN & BARLEY SOUP

This is one of Milly's favourite store cupboard midweek suppers. It's pure comfort food. Do make sure you use good stock for this as it's such an important component in the final flavour. Great topped with Parmesan or pecorino.

SERVES 4

1 tablespoon rapeseed oil
2 onions, finely chopped
1 garlic clove, crushed
2 celery sticks, chopped
1 fennel bulb, cored and chopped
50g (¼ cup) pearl barley
1 bay leaf
1.2–1.5 litres (5–6 cups) good vegetable stock
150g (2 cups) baby spinach, roughly chopped
400g (14oz) can butterbeans, drained and rinsed
400g (14oz) can flageolet beans, drained and rinsed
sea salt and black pepper
75g (2½oz) pecorino or Parmesan
dill sprigs, to serve

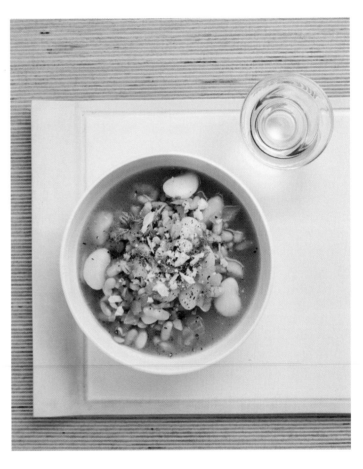

Heat the oil in a large saucepan and gently sauté the onions, garlic, celery and fennel until lovely and tender – about 15 minutes. If the veggies are catching a little, add a splash of water.

Stir in the pearl barley, bay leaf and 1.2 litres (5 cups) of the stock and bring to the boil. Simmer for 40 minutes until the pearl barley is tender, giving an occasional stir as you pass by.

Stir in the spinach and beans and heat to wilt the spinach. Season to taste and add more stock to thin down the soup if you like.

Ladle into bowls and serve with the pecorino or Parmesan, grated straight over the top, and a sprinkling of dill.

# MY FAVOURITE FISH CHOWDER

SERVES 4

I use frozen fish for this, popped straight from the freezer into the simmering soup.
I adore smoked haddock but it works brilliantly with cod and jumbo prawns too.

1 tablespoon olive oil
2 onions, finely chopped
2 carrots, finely chopped
2 celery sticks, finely chopped
2 parsnips, finely chopped
4 slices of lean prosciutto
800ml–1 litre (3¼–4 cups) good fish stock
200g (7oz) chunky white fish fillets, cubed
200g (7oz) undyed smoked haddock, cubed
200g (7oz) can sweetcorn, drained
100g (⅓ cup) low-fat Greek yogurt
2 tablespoons chopped chives
sea salt and black pepper

Heat the olive oil in a large saucepan over
a medium heat and sweat the onions, carrots,
celery and parsnips until tender, about
10 minutes.

Meanwhile, heat a dry frying pan over medium
heat. Add the prosciutto slices and fry until
crispy. Lay on some kitchen paper to drain.

Add the stock to the veggie pan and bring
to the boil. Turn down the heat and add the
fish, simmering gently for 3–5 minutes until
cooked through. Stir through the sweetcorn
and Greek yogurt and season to taste.

Ladle into bowls and top each portion with
chives and crispy prosciutto pieces.

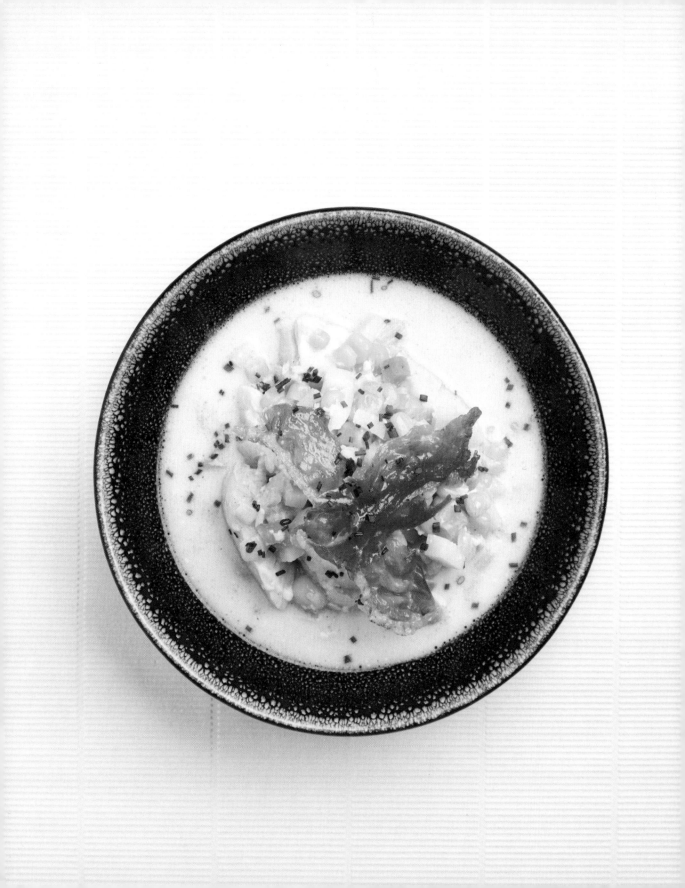

# CHICKEN 'RAMEN' SOUP

Leftover roast chicken is perfect for this, but you can use raw chicken instead. Simply poach in the simmering stock for 10–15 minutes until cooked through, then let it cool in the stock before shredding. If you don't have a spiralizer, use a julienne or normal vegetable peeler.

SERVES 4

1.5 litres (6 cups) good chicken stock

2 tablespoons peeled and grated fresh root ginger

1 red chilli, sliced

2 tablespoons reduced-sodium soy sauce

large handful of fresh coriander, leaves and stalks chopped separately

125g (4½oz) shiitake mushrooms, sliced

200g (7oz) pak choi, stalks and leaves chopped separately

4 large carrots, spiralized into 'noodles'

200g (7oz) cooked chicken, shredded

4 medium eggs, hard boiled, peeled and halved

2 spring onions, finely sliced

2 teaspoons black sesame seeds

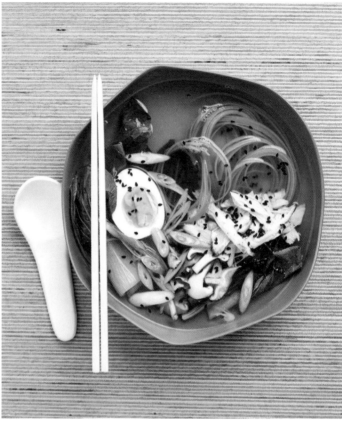

Place the chicken stock in a large saucepan with the ginger, chilli, soy sauce and coriander stems and heat until boiling. Bubble for a few minutes to help intensify the flavour.

Add the mushrooms, pak choi stalks and spiralized carrots to the simmering stock and cook for a couple of minutes until just tender. Finally, stir in the chicken and pak choi leaves to heat through and check for seasoning, adjusting with a little more soy sauce if you like.

Ladle into bowls and top with coriander leaves, boiled egg halves, spring onions and sesame seeds to serve.

Meanwhile, mix all the salsa ingredients in a large bowl and season to taste. Serve with the griddled chicken, with some lime wedges to squeeze over.

# MUMMY'S MULLIGATAWNY ⓥ

Usually made with rice, but I've swapped in chickpeas for a higher protein content. I've had kids on sleepovers have seconds of this, so do dish it up for kids with wholemeal pitta chips.

2 tablespoons butter
1 tablespoon vegetable oil
1 onion, chopped
2 garlic cloves, crushed
3 carrots, chopped
3 celery sticks, sliced
1 apple, peeled, cored and chopped
½ tablespoon curry powder
1 tablespoon tomato purée
1 litre (4 cups) good vegetable stock
½ teaspoon sea salt
½ teaspoon black pepper
400g (14oz) can chickpeas, drained and rinsed
100g (⅓ cup) low-fat Greek yogurt
handful of flat leaf parsley leaves, chopped
50g (⅔ cup) toasted flaked almonds

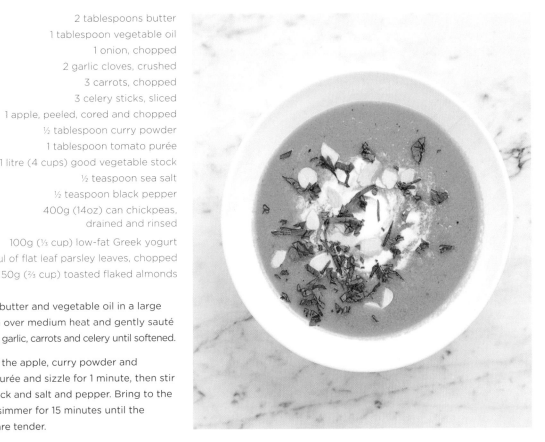

Heat the butter and vegetable oil in a large saucepan over medium heat and gently sauté the onion, garlic, carrots and celery until softened.

Now add the apple, curry powder and tomato purée and sizzle for 1 minute, then stir in the stock and salt and pepper. Bring to the boil and simmer for 15 minutes until the veggies are tender.

Transfer, in batches, to a high-speed blender and give it a really good whizz until extra smooth. Have a taste to check if the seasoning is right for you.

Return to the pan, stir in the chickpeas and reheat the soup. Ladle into bowls and serve with a dollop of yogurt to stir through and a sprinkle of the parsley and almonds.

# CHOI SUM BEEF SOUP

Don't be put off by the long ingredients list – it's a doddle to make and delicious. I prep the soup while Paul fries up the steak and we add the chilli at the table. The girls put out little bowls of Thai basil, extra onion, chopped cashews, extra lime and chopsticks.

2 x 150g (5½oz) fillet steaks

700ml (scant 3 cups) good beef stock

1 red onion, finely sliced

1 tablespoon peeled and grated
fresh root ginger

1 star anise

1 small cinnamon stick

1 tablespoon reduced-sodium soy sauce

1 teaspoon groundnut oil

100g (3½oz) choi sum, chopped

100g (3½oz) sugar snap peas

small handful of Thai basil leaves, sliced

juice of ½ lime

½ red chilli, sliced

2 spring onions, halved and finely
shredded lengthways

lime wedges, to serve

Remove the steaks from the fridge and allow them to come to room temperature before cooking.

Place the beef stock in a large saucepan with the onion, ginger, star anise, cinnamon stick and soy sauce. Bring to the boil, then bubble for a few minutes to help intensify the flavour.

Heat the oil in a frying pan over high heat and add the steaks. Cook for 2–5 minutes on each side, depending on how well cooked you like them. Cooking time will also depend on the cut: the thicker the cut, the longer you will need to cook the meat. Season the steaks and set aside, covered in foil, for at least 5 minutes to rest.

Add the choi sum and sugar snap peas to the hot stock and simmer until the veggies are tender but still have a little bite to them. Stir in the Thai basil and lime juice. Taste for seasoning, adding a little more soy sauce if you like.

Lift out the cinnamon stick and star anise and ladle the soup into bowls. Slice the steak and add to the soup, then sprinkle over the red chilli and spring onions. I like mine with extra zing so I serve the soup with lime wedges.

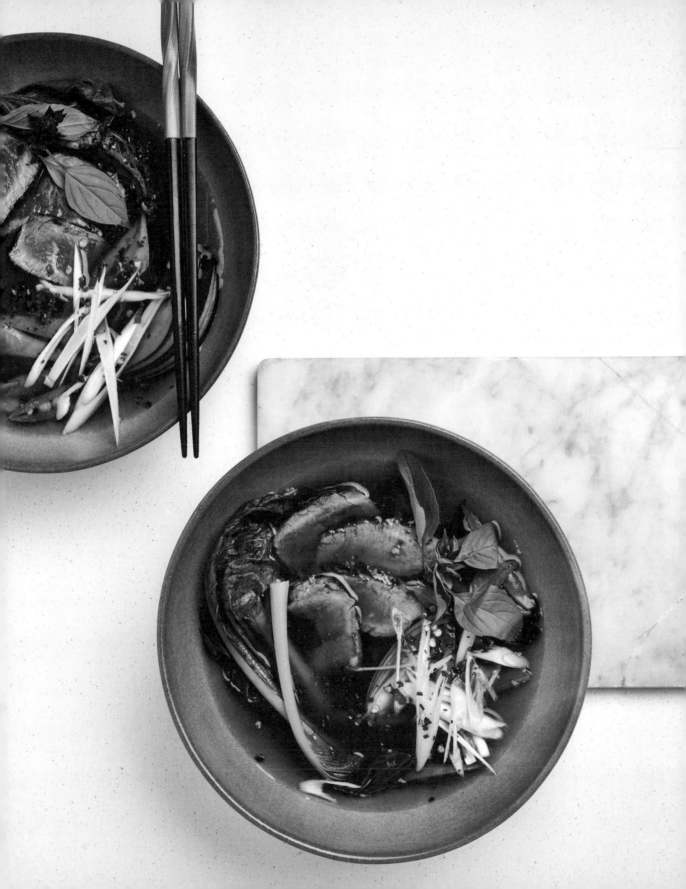

# TOFU, BUTTERBEAN & KALE SOUP (Vg)

Vegan comfort soup at its best. Works wonderfully with spring greens too, or a few frozen peas thrown in. Try it with smoked tofu also for added flavour.

SERVES 4

400g (14oz) firm tofu, cubed
1½ tablespoons rapeseed oil
1 onion, finely sliced
1 leek, sliced
2 garlic cloves, crushed
1 teaspoon smoked sweet paprika
75g (2¾oz) curly kale, coarse stems discarded, torn into bite-sized pieces
400g (14oz) can chopped tomatoes
200ml (scant 1 cup) good vegetable stock
½ teaspoon sea salt
¼ teaspoon black pepper
400g (14oz) can butterbeans, drained and rinsed

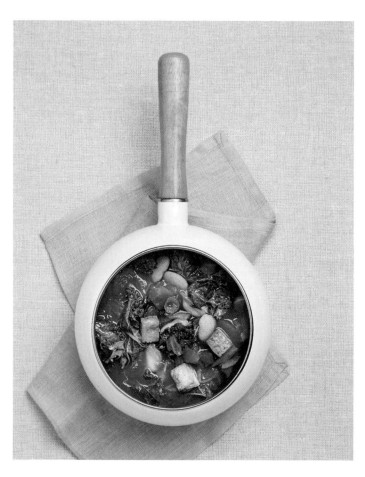

Blot the tofu dry with kitchen paper. Heat 1 tablespoon of the rapeseed oil in a large nonstick saucepan over medium heat. Add the tofu and brown on all sides, turning carefully. Remove from the pan and set aside.

Heat the remaining oil in the saucepan and gently sauté the onion, leek and garlic for 5 minutes. Stir in the smoked paprika and kale, adding a splash of water to help steam-fry the kale. Cook for 2–3 minutes then stir in the tomatoes, stock, salt and pepper.

Simmer for about 5 minutes until the kale is cooked to your liking. I like it relatively well cooked, but go with your preference.

Carefully stir in the butterbeans and tofu, trying not to break up the tofu, and season to taste. It's ready to serve up.

# BROCCOLI, CAULIFLOWER & PANEER CURRY ⓥ

In the Lifestyle Phase I make this with full-fat cheese and serve with a side of yogurt, cucumber topped with mustard seeds and warm wholemeal roti. It's a great dish for family suppers.

SERVES 4

1 tablespoon groundnut oil
225g (8oz) paneer cheese, cubed
100g (⅓ cup) cauliflower florets
100g (½ cup) broccoli florets
2 onions, finely sliced
1 garlic clove, crushed
1 tablespoon mild curry paste
100ml (scant ½ cup) good vegetable stock
500g (2 cups) passata or sieved tomatoes
200g (7oz) frozen chopped spinach
2 tablespoons unsweetened desiccated coconut, plus extra to sprinkle
175g (¾ cup) low-fat Greek yogurt
2 spring onions, finely sliced
sea salt and black pepper

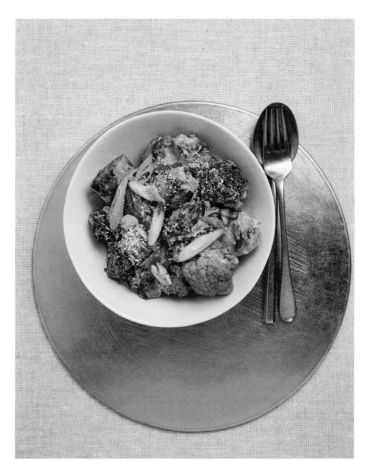

Heat the oil in a large deep frying pan over medium-high heat and brown the paneer on all sides. Remove from the pan and set aside.

Next add the cauliflower and broccoli to the pan and sauté until beginning to colour, then turn down the heat a little and add the onions. Fry for a couple of minutes, stirring, to soften before adding the garlic, curry paste and stock. Cook for a few seconds.

Pour in the passata and mix in the spinach and coconut. Bring to the boil and simmer for 10 minutes until the veggies are tender and the sauce has thickened.

Stir in the yogurt and paneer. Heat through and season to taste. Sprinkle over the spring onions and a little more coconut and it's ready for serving.

# CHICKEN & CHICKPEA TAGINE

I love the sweetness of a Moroccan tagine. They are usually made with dried fruit, which is high in sugar, so I've swapped in some fresh mango at the end to replicate that fruity tang.

SERVES 2

1 tablespoon olive oil
2 onions, finely sliced
2 garlic cloves, crushed
1 teaspoon harissa paste
1 teaspoon ground cinnamon
½ teaspoon ground cumin
350g (12oz) skinless boneless chicken thighs, sliced
200g (⅔ cup) cauliflower florets
2 x 400g (14oz) cans chopped tomatoes
250ml (1 cup) good chicken stock
½ teaspoon sea salt
1 teaspoon black pepper
400g (14oz) can chickpeas, drained and rinsed
¼ ripe mango, finely chopped
75g (generous 1 cup) baby spinach
large handful of coriander leaves, chopped

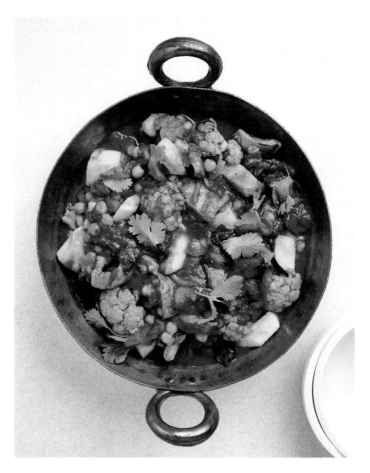

Heat the oil in a large saucepan over medium-low heat and cook the onions for 10 minutes until golden and translucent. Add the garlic, harissa and spices and sizzle for a few seconds before stirring in the chicken and cauliflower florets.

Mix to coat, then add the tomatoes, stock, salt and pepper. Bring to the boil and simmer for 15 minutes until the sauce has thickened.

Stir in the chickpeas, mango and spinach, stirring until the leaves wilt. Taste for seasoning, adjusting as you like. Spoon into bowls and scatter over the coriander to serve.

# MONDAY CHICKEN STEW

Great for Monday night suppers after a Sunday roast chicken. I boil up the stock on Sunday night and add in leftover chicken in the final stage to heat through. Any bean will do.

1 garlic clove, finely sliced
1 leek, finely sliced
2 celery sticks, sliced
1 carrot, finely chopped
300g (10½oz) skinless boneless chicken thighs or breast, cut into chunks
100g (⅔ cup) green beans, chopped
leaves from ½ thyme sprig
400g (14oz) can haricot beans, drained and rinsed
500–750ml (2–3 cups) good chicken or vegetable stock
small handful of flat leaf parsley, chopped
sea salt and black pepper

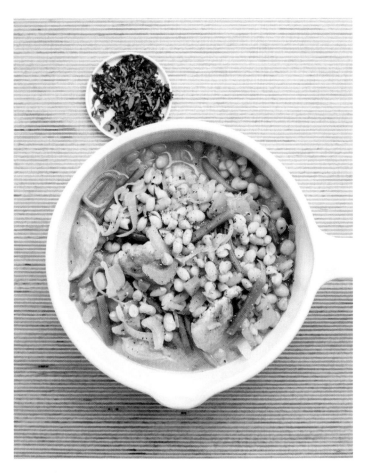

Heat the oil in a large saucepan and add the garlic, leek, celery and carrot. Sauté for 5 minutes over a medium heat until the leeks are transparent.

Add the chicken, green beans and thyme and fry for a few more minutes to get some colour on the chicken.

Next add the haricot beans and pour in 500ml (2 cups) of the stock, stirring to remove all the good brown bits from the base of the pan. Bring to the boil, then reduce the heat and simmer for a few minutes, just until the chicken is cooked through but the veggies still have a little bite to them.

Stir through the parsley and season to taste, adding a little more stock if you'd like a thinner sauce. Serve the stew in bowls.

# WARM WHITE MISO & TOFU SALAD (Vg)

This is so simple and so delicious. If you can't find white miso, you can use a little English mustard. Just a little cornflour helps the tofu crisp up beautifully.

¾ cucumber, finely sliced into rounds
½ teaspoon sea salt
200g (7oz) piece of firm tofu, cut into fingers
1 tablespoon cornflour
1 tablespoon groundnut oil
2 carrots, peeled into ribbons
1 green pepper, cored, deseeded and sliced
2 spring onions, sliced
handful of flat leaf parsley leaves, chopped
25g (⅓ cup) unsalted cashew nuts, chopped
1 teaspoon poppy seeds

### FOR THE DRESSING
¼ teaspoon white miso paste
1 tablespoon groundnut oil
large pinch of dried chilli flakes
juice of ½ lemon

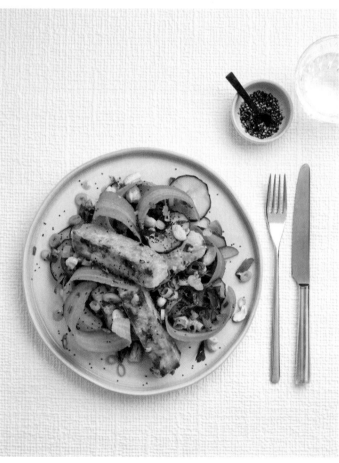

Put the cucumber into a colander in the sink and sprinkle over the salt. Leave for 10 minutes, tossing occasionally, to draw water from it for a more crunchy texture.

Blot the tofu dry with kitchen paper and coat with the cornflour. Heat the oil in a nonstick frying pan over medium heat and cook the tofu fingers, turning gently, until browned and crispy on the outside. Set aside.

Tip the cucumber onto a few sheets of kitchen paper and pat dry. Empty into a large bowl and mix in the carrots, pepper, spring onions, parsley, cashew nuts and poppy seeds.

Mix the dressing ingredients together, then mix into the salad. Serve in shallow bowls, topped with the crispy tofu.

# SALMON & SESAME GREENS

This is super-speedy and the greens are the star, so full of flavour. This works just as well with chicken, tofu or steak – ring the changes.

SERVES 2

1 tablespoon groundnut oil
2 x 150g (5½oz) skinless salmon fillets
1 teaspoon white miso paste
200g (7oz) Tenderstem broccoli
200g (7oz) asparagus tips
½ Chinese leaf cabbage, shredded
1 tablespoon peeled and grated
fresh root ginger
2 garlic cloves, finely sliced
1 tablespoon white wine vinegar
2 tablespoons reduced-sodium soy sauce
1 teaspoon toasted sesame oil
½ tablespoon black sesame seeds

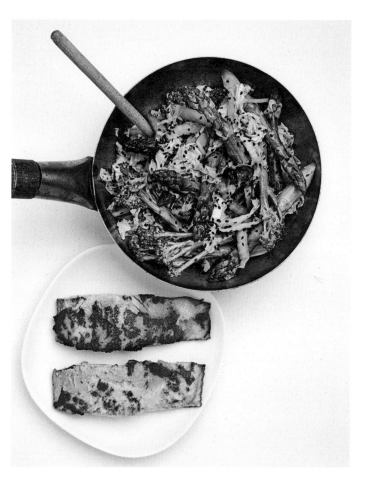

Heat 1 teaspoon of the groundnut oil in a wok over low-medium heat. Brush the salmon fillets with the miso paste and cook for 5 minutes, turning once. I like them a little charred but still juicy on the inside. Lift onto a plate and cover with foil to keep warm.

Turn up the heat and add the remaining oil to the pan. Stir-fry the broccoli for 2 minutes, adding a splash of water to help it cook. Next add the asparagus, shredded Chinese leaf, ginger and garlic and continue to stir-fry until the veggies are tender but still have some bite to them.

Add the vinegar, soy sauce and toasted sesame oil and toss together well.

Serve in shallow bowls topped with the salmon and the sesame seeds.

# ROCKET, FISH & CANNELLINI STEW

This is a stew but it's so light and speedy that it's a great dish for summer evenings too. Its simplicity really shows off all the ingredients. It goes well with all firm white fish, or serve with grilled chicken breasts if you prefer.

SERVES 2

1 tablespoon rapeseed oil
1 leek, thickly sliced
1 garlic clove, finely sliced
1 rosemary sprig
300–500ml (1¼–2 cups) good fish stock
400g (14oz) can cannellini beans, drained and rinsed
2 x 125g (4½oz) cod fillets
finely grated zest and juice of ½ lemon
50g (1¾oz) rocket, chopped
2 teaspoons good-quality pesto
2 tablespoons chopped flat leaf parsley leaves
sea salt and black pepper

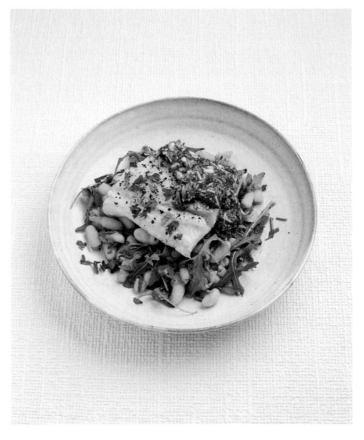

Preheat the grill to medium.

Heat the oil in a large nonstick saucepan and gently cook the leek for 10 minutes until tender and translucent; make sure it is soft as tough leeks aren't pleasant. Add a splash of water occasionally to help it along.

Stir in the garlic, rosemary, stock and cannellini beans and bring to the boil.

Lay the fish on a baking tray, season to taste and grill for 5 minutes until cooked through.

Add the lemon zest and juice and the rocket to the saucepan and cook gently until the rocket has wilted. Season to taste and pick out the rosemary sprig. Spoon the stew into shallow bowls and top with the fish. Spoon over the pesto, sprinkle on the parsley and serve.

# CURRIED COD WITH PUY LENTILS & SPINACH

Pre-cooked lentils are a speedy and nutritious store cupboard standby which I often reach for. But you can of course cook your own – just remember to give them a good rinse in cold water before simmering in stock or water until tender.

2 teaspoons mild curry paste
2 x 125g (4½oz) skinless cod fillets
small knob of butter
1 teaspoon groundnut oil

### FOR THE LENTILS
1 teaspoon groundnut oil
1 garlic clove, crushed
½ teaspoon ground cumin
½ red chilli, chopped
150g (1¼ cups) cherry tomatoes
250g (9oz) pouch or can of
ready-to-eat Puy lentils
100ml (scant ½ cup) good fish stock
50g (⅔ cup) baby spinach
1 tablespoon red wine vinegar
sea salt and black pepper

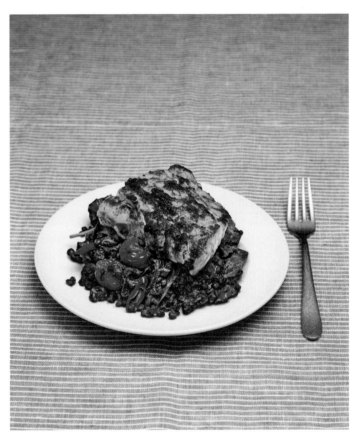

For the lentils, heat the oil in a large frying pan and sizzle the garlic, cumin, chilli and tomatoes for 1 minute until they smell fragrant.

Stir in the lentils and stock and season to taste. Cook until the pan is nearly dry and the tomatoes are just catching.

Meanwhile, brush the curry paste over the fish. Heat the butter and oil in a nonstick frying pan over medium-high heat until the butter is foaming. Cook the fish for 3–5 minutes, turning once, until cooked through.

Stir the spinach and vinegar into the warm lentils to wilt the leaves and taste for seasoning, adjusting as you like. Serve the fish on top of the lentils.

# MAYNARD CHICKEN & MUSTARD BURGERS

Once cooked and cooled, these tasty burgers freeze well and make a great addition to any salad. For a nut-free version, use a slice of wholemeal bread, whizzed into breadcrumbs, instead of the ground almonds. If you can, make the slaw a day ahead to let the flavours mingle. Cover and keep in the fridge, then mix again before serving.

SERVES 4

3 skinless chicken breasts, about 150g (5½oz) each

½ tablespoon wholegrain mustard

finely grated zest of ½ lemon

large handful of flat leaf parsley, chopped

1 tablespoon chopped tarragon leaves

1 egg

3 tablespoons ground almonds

½ teaspoon sea salt

1 teaspoon olive oil

FOR THE SLAW

juice of ½–1 lemon

2 tablespoons good-quality hummus

100g (⅓ cup) low-fat Greek yogurt

½ small red cabbage, cored and finely shredded

2 carrots, coarsely grated or spiralized

good handful of flat leaf parsley, chopped

¼ red onion, finely chopped

1 apple, peeled, cored and chopped

sea salt and black pepper

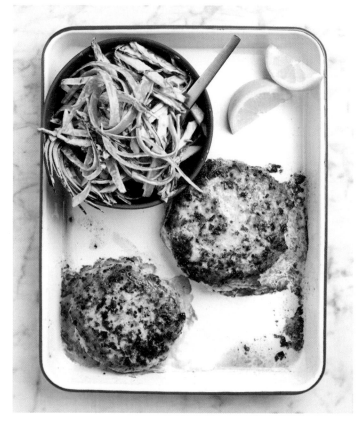

Preheat the oven to 200°C/400°F/Gas Mark 6.

For the burgers, whizz the chicken in a food processor until finely chopped. Add the mustard, lemon zest, parsley, tarragon, egg, almonds and salt and whizz again to combine. Shape into 4 flattened patties, cover and chill for 20 minutes to firm up and help them stay together when cooked.

Meanwhile make the slaw. Mix the lemon juice, hummus and yogurt in a large bowl and add the remaining slaw ingredients. Season to taste, toss in the dressing and add some more lemon juice if you like.

Heat the oil in a large nonstick frying pan and cook the chicken burgers for 5 minutes, turning once, until golden all over. If the pan is ovenproof, pop it straight into the oven for 15 minutes until the burgers are cooked through. Alternatively, transfer them to a baking tray first. Frying the burgers first, then finishing them off in the oven, keeps them extra juicy.

Serve the burgers with the slaw.

# RUBY CHICKEN QUINOA

Marinade the breasts for the tenderest of chicken. The pretty quinoa salad is a hit with my girls and we'll often have it as a meal on its own with crumbled feta cheese. The sweet and salty tang works a treat and is great for weekday lunchboxes

SERVES 2

2 skinless chicken breasts, about 150g (5½oz) each
1 tablespoon aged balsamic vinegar
2 tablespoons tomato purée
½ teaspoon ground cinnamon
1 teaspoon olive oil
sea salt and black pepper

FOR THE QUINOA
100g (½ cup) quinoa
75g (2¾oz) pomegranate seeds
small handful of coriander leaves, chopped
small handful of mint leaves, chopped
1 teaspoon lime juice
25g (scant ¼ cup) unsalted pistachios, chopped
1 spring onion, finely sliced
1 tablespoon extra virgin olive oil
75g (2¾oz) feta, crumbled

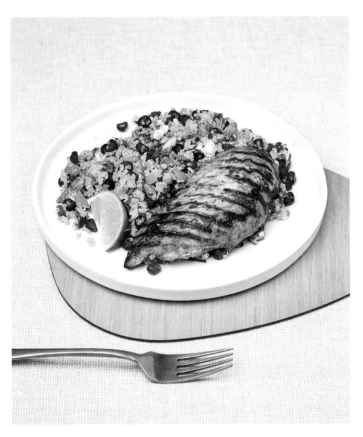

Place the chicken into a sandwich bag or non-metallic bowl with the vinegar, tomato purée and cinnamon and season to taste. Close (or cover) and leave to marinate in the fridge for 30 minutes, or overnight if you want to get ahead. Sometimes, if I'm really pushed for time, I leave out the marinating time.

Cook the quinoa in a saucepan of salted boiling water until tender – this takes about 15 minutes. Drain well then empty into a large bowl and mix in the remaining quinoa ingredients; the warm quinoa will suck up all the flavours. Season to taste.

Heat the oil in a nonstick griddle pan and pop in the chicken. Griddle, turning occasionally, until the chicken is beautifully stripy on both sides and cooked through – about 10 minutes in total.

Slice the chicken and serve on top of the quinoa salad.

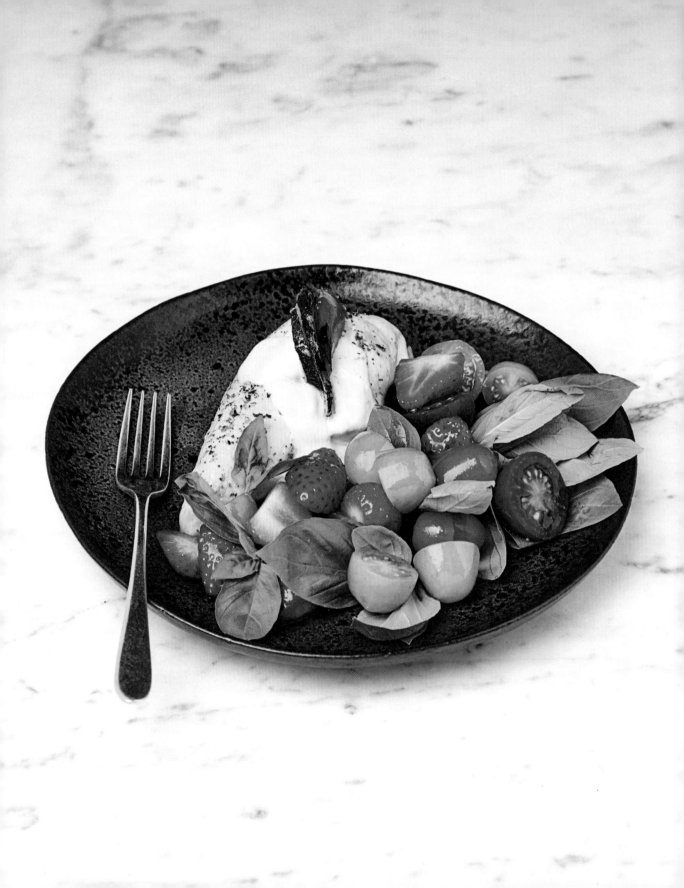

# PRIMAVERA CHICKEN WITH STRAWBERRY SALAD

I cook primavera chicken so often for my daughters, with all sorts of sides, but in summer I love using the ripest of strawberries and tomatoes for this weird but wonderful salad. It's all about good ingredients.

4 skinless chicken breasts, about 150g (5½oz) each

1 red onion, peeled
handful of basil leaves
1 courgette, finely sliced into rounds
1 red pepper, cored, deseeded and sliced
1½ teaspoons dried mixed herbs
¼ teaspoon sea salt
¼ teaspoon black pepper
100g (3½oz) mozzarella, chopped

## FOR THE SALAD

4 tomatoes, a mix of colours if you can find them, chopped

200g (1 cup) ripe strawberries, chopped
large handful of basil leaves, sliced
1 tablespoon aged balsamic vinegar

Preheat the oven to 200°C/400°F/Gas Mark 6.

Cut 4 slits, evenly spaced, into the top of each chicken breast. You want to cut about halfway down into the meat. Arrange the chicken in an ovenproof dish with the cuts facing upwards.

Cut the onion into 16 wedges (don't cut too much off the root end as this holds the wedges together nicely). Stuff a wedge of onion, a slice each of courgette and pepper and a basil leaf into each of the slits in the chicken breasts. Don't worry if you can't get them all in, just get in as much as you can and try to make them look pretty!

Sprinkle over the mixed herbs, salt, pepper and mozzarella. Bake for 25 minutes until the chicken is cooked through.

Meanwhile mix all the salad ingredients together, season to taste and toss well. Serve with the stuffed chicken.

# CHICKEN TIKKA MASALA WITH SPINACH & CHICKPEAS

I love the full flavour and juiciness of chicken thighs, but use skinless chicken breast if you prefer. To defrost your spinach quickly, cover it with boiling water. After draining (and cooling a little), give it a good squeeze to get rid of the extra water.

SERVES 4

1 tablespoon groundnut oil
2 onions, finely sliced
2 garlic cloves, crushed
2 courgettes, coarsely grated
2 tablespoons tikka masala paste
500g (1lb 2oz) skinless boneless chicken thighs, sliced
400g (14oz) can chopped tomatoes
125g (1 cup) frozen peas
100g (⅓ cup) low-fat Greek yogurt
½ teaspoon sea salt
leaves from 1 bunch of coriander, chopped (optional

### FOR THE SPINACH
1 tablespoon groundnut oil
2 garlic cloves, crushed
250g (9oz) frozen leaf spinach, defrosted
400g (14oz) can chickpeas, drained and rinsed
squeeze of lemon juice
sea salt and black pepper

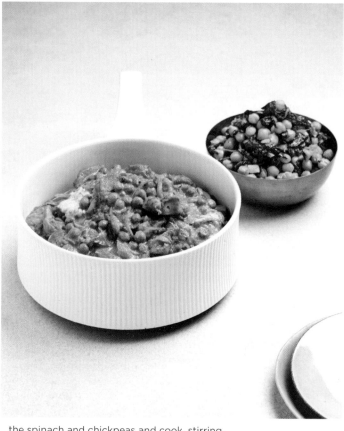

Heat the oil in a large deep frying pan over low-medium heat and cook the onions, stirring often, until they are golden. Add a splash of water to the pan if they are beginning to catch.

Add the garlic, courgettes, spice paste and chicken (I have a trusty pair of kitchen scissors which I deploy for snipping the chicken straight into the pan). Fry, stirring from time to time, until really lovely and aromatic. Add the tomatoes and cook for 15 minutes.

For the spinach, heat the oil in a wok and sizzle the garlic for a few seconds. Add

the spinach and chickpeas and cook, stirring, until piping hot. Add a squeeze of lemon and season to taste, then keep warm while you finish off the curry.

Add the peas, Greek yogurt and salt to the curry and simmer for a couple of minutes to let the flavours mingle and the peas defrost. Sprinkle the curry with plenty of coriander, if liked, and serve with the spinach.

# LAMB CURRY WITH SPICED CAULIFLOWER RICE

This is my go-to-in-a-hurry curry. Because the lamb leg steaks are relatively lean, they don't need slow cooking. Turmeric and black onion seeds are what make this cauliflower rice such a nice accompaniment to any curry.

SERVES 4

1 tablespoon groundnut oil
2 onions, finely sliced
2 carrots, finely diced
2 garlic cloves, crushed
1 tablespoon peeled and grated fresh root ginger
1 red chilli, chopped
1 teaspoon ground cumin
1 teaspoon ground coriander
400g (14oz) lamb leg steaks (visible fat trimmed), cubed
2 x 400g (14oz) cans chopped tomatoes
25g (scant ¼ cup) toasted flaked almonds
sea salt and black pepper

### FOR THE CAULIFLOWER RICE
1 large cauliflower, cut into florets (about 700g/1lb 9oz)
1 teaspoon black onion seeds
¼ teaspoon ground turmeric

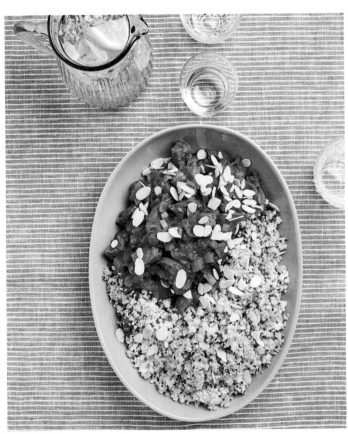

Heat the oil in a large deep frying pan over low-medium heat and cook the onions and carrots, stirring often, until they are golden (have patience, softened onions are the base of a good curry). Add the garlic, ginger, chilli and ground spices and fry for 1 minute.

Add the lamb to the pan and cook for a couple of minutes to brown the meat. Then add the chopped tomatoes and simmer for 15 minutes.

Meanwhile, pulse the cauliflower in a food processor until it looks like rice. Heat a splash of water in a large frying pan over high heat.

Add the cauliflower, black onion seeds and turmeric and cook for about 5 minutes until tender, adding a splash more water if needed. Season to taste.

Season the lamb curry, scatter over the almonds and serve with the cauliflower rice.

# EMMA'S SPRING COD EN PAPILLOTE

SERVES 4

I love cooking en papillote as the food cooks in its own steam, keeping it so juicy and flavoursome. You can make the parcels up to 30 minutes ahead, but any more and the paper can get quite soggy. Raw courgette has a lovely mild flavour and good crunch, ideal for a salad.

200g (1½ cups) cherry tomatoes, mixed colours if possible

150g (1 cup) mangetout

2 carrots, cut into matchsticks

2 x 125g (4½oz) skinless cod fillets

1 tablespoon chopped oregano leaves, or 1 teaspoon dried oregano

1 tablespoon capers, rinsed

2 lemons

2 tablespoons extra virgin olive oil

sea salt and black pepper

FOR THE SALAD

3 courgettes

leaves from 1 bunch of basil, torn

1 tablespoon extra virgin olive oil

1 teaspoon wholegrain mustard

100g (3½oz) feta, crumbled

50g (scant ½ cup) unsalted pistachios, chopped

Preheat the oven to 200°C/400°F/Gas Mark 6.

Cut 4 large squares of baking paper. Fold each in half, make a crease, open out again and lay them out on your work surface. Make a mound of veggies on one side of each piece of paper. Lay the fish on top of the veggies, sprinkle over the oregano and capers and season to taste. Now squeeze the juice of ½ lemon on to each pile and drizzle over the oil.

Fold the other half of the paper over the fish and, starting at one end, make a series of small tight folds all the way around the open edge, working into the fish, sealing it in. You should end up with a crimped effect all the way round the edges, apart from the fold.

Carefully lift the parcels onto a baking tray and cook in the oven for 20 minutes.

Meanwhile, use a vegetable peeler to peel the courgettes into ribbons, discarding the inner seedy core. Put into a large bowl with the basil, oil and mustard. Season to taste, toss to coat, then gently mix in the feta and pistachios. Set aside.

Take the parcels, still sealed, to the table and serve with the courgette salad. Be careful when you open the parcels as the steam will be hot.

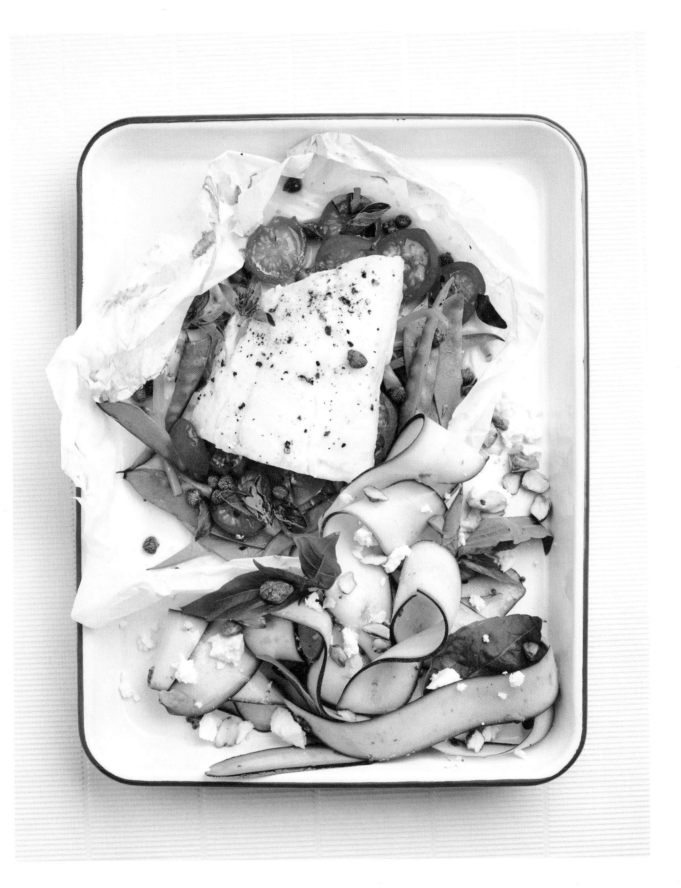

# MR P'S TUNA BURGERS

My husband's tuna patties are divine. They adapt well with a little Thai green curry paste and Thai basil, and served with any side. This orange and avo salad works well with my sesame tuna steaks too (see *The Louise Parker Method: Lean for Life*, page 128).

SERVES 2

250g (9oz) yellow fin tuna steaks
2 spring onions, chopped
small handful of basil leaves
2 teaspoons capers, rinsed
finely grated zest of ½ lemon
1 tablespoon olive oil
sea salt and black pepper

### FOR THE SALAD
1 orange
pinch of dried chilli flakes
2 tomatoes, chopped
finely grated zest and juice of ½ lime
small handful of parsley leaves, finely chopped
1 ripe avocado, chopped

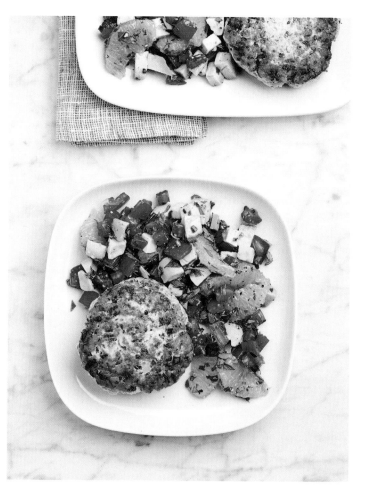

Put the tuna into a food processor with the spring onions, basil, capers and lemon zest, season to taste and whizz until finely chopped and coming together. Shape into 4 flattened patties, cover and chill for 10 minutes to firm up.

Meanwhile, peel and slice the orange, removing as much pith as possible, then cut the slices into quarters. Put into a bowl and mix in the chilli flakes, tomatoes, lime zest and juice and parsley. Season to taste and carefully mix through the avocado. Set aside.

Heat the oil in a large nonstick frying pan and fry the tuna burgers for 10 minutes, turning once, until cooked through. Serve the burgers with the salad.

# SUNSHINE FISH STEW

This warms up any winter night and works well with any firm white fish. Use good-quality Italian tinned tomatoes and you can leave out the chilli if you're cooking for young kids. The lentils make a hearty meal of it and soak up all the flavours.

SERVES 4

1 tablespoon olive oil
1 red onion, finely sliced
1 red pepper, cored, deseeded and chopped
1 orange pepper, cored, deseeded and chopped
1 teaspoon sweet smoked paprika
¼–½ teaspoon dried chilli flakes
1 thyme sprig
100g (½ cup) dried red lentils, rinsed in cold water
2 x 400g (14oz) cans chopped tomatoes
250ml (1 cup) good fish stock
½ teaspoon sea salt
½ teaspoon black pepper
350g (12oz) white fish fillets, cubed
125g (4½oz) peeled king prawns, deveined
large handful of flat leaf parsley leaves, chopped
lime wedges, to serve

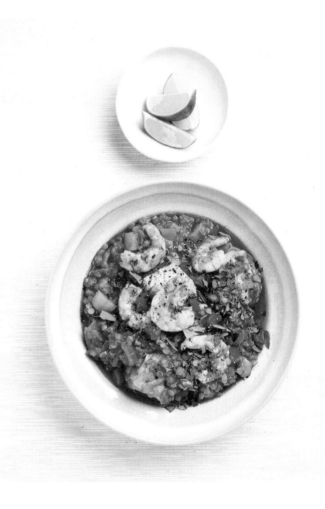

Heat the olive oil in a large saucepan over medium heat and sauté the onion until softened. Add the peppers and fry to soften slightly. Stir in the paprika, chilli, thyme and lentils and fry for a minute or two to get the flavours going.

Now add the tomatoes, stock, salt and pepper and bring to the boil. Cook for 15 minutes until the lentils and veggies are tender.

Submerge the fish and prawns into the stew and simmer gently until they are just cooked through. Finally, taste for seasoning, adjusting if needed.

Sprinkle over the parsley and serve the stew with lime wedges on the side.

# GRIDDLED STEAK WITH CAPONATA & ROASTED BROCCOLI

SERVES 2

You can use any steak here – sirloin, fillet, ribeye, or the very trendy bavette which is rammed with flavour and still great value. Alternatively, griddled chicken breast or halloumi both work a treat. Traditionally caponata is made with raisins, but I've added some fresh grapes for that hint of sweetness. This caponata improves with age so keep a batch in the fridge and eat at room temperature or gently warm through for an instant meal.

2 x 150g (5½oz) fillet steaks
1 teaspoon olive oil
sea salt and black pepper

FOR THE CAPONATA
1 teaspoon olive oil
2 shallots, finely sliced
1 aubergine, chopped
400g (14oz) can cherry tomatoes
1 tablespoon capers, rinsed
1 tablespoon toasted pine nuts
1 tablespoon red wine vinegar
10 red seedless grapes, halved
handful of basil leaves

FOR THE BROCCOLI
200g (generous 1 cup) broccoli florets
1 tablespoon olive oil
1 garlic clove, crushed
25g (¼ cup) finely grated Parmesan

Preheat oven to 200°C/400°F/Gas Mark 6.

Remove the steaks from the fridge and allow to come to room temperature before cooking.

For the caponata, heat the oil in a large nonstick saucepan over medium heat. Add the shallots and aubergine and cook until tender – this can take a while as aubergines are stubborn, but give them time and they'll reward you! Add a little splash of water to the pan if it looks like the aubergines are catching. Now stir in the remaining caponata ingredients except for the basil and simmer for 10 minutes. Don't forget to taste for seasoning.

Meanwhile, toss the broccoli florets, olive oil and garlic on a small baking tray and season to taste. Spread them out and bake for 10–15 minutes until they are crispy at the edges and the stalks are just tender.

Heat the oil in a frying pan over high heat and add the steaks. Cook for 2–5 minutes on each side, depending on how well cooked you like them. Cooking time will also depend on the cut: the thicker the cut, the longer you will need to cook the meat. Season the steaks and set aside, covered in foil, for at least 5 minutes to rest.

Toss the cheese through the broccoli and stir the basil through the caponata. Serve both with the rested steaks.

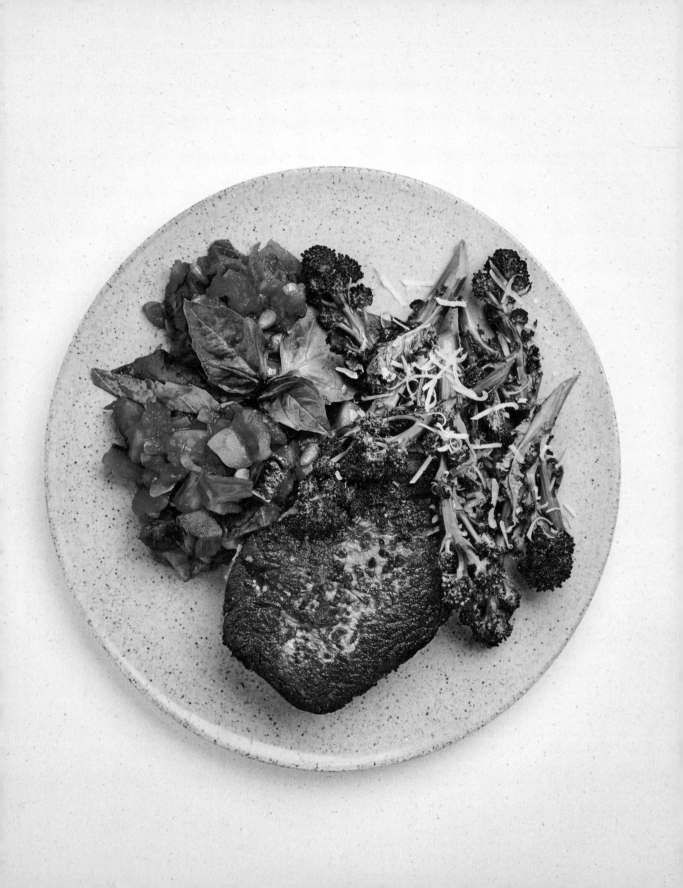

# MEXICAN CHICKEN & SALSA

Great for griddling and barbecuing. You can roast your own peppers for 20–25 minutes in a very hot oven. Once cooled a little, squeeze out the pips and liquid, remove the skin and roughly chop the flesh.

SERVES 2

2 skinless chicken breasts, about 150g (5½oz) each

2 tablespoons tomato purée
1 teaspoon chipotle paste
finely grated zest of 1 lime
1 teaspoon olive oil
sea salt and black pepper
lime wedges, to serve

FOR THE SALSA
2 whole roasted peppers from a jar, drained and chopped

150g (1¼ cups) cherry tomatoes, halved
400g (14oz) can black-eyed beans, drained and rinsed

100g (scant ½ cup) sweetcorn kernels
½ red onion, finely sliced
1 red chilli, sliced
juice of 1 lime
leaves from 1 bunch of coriander, chopped

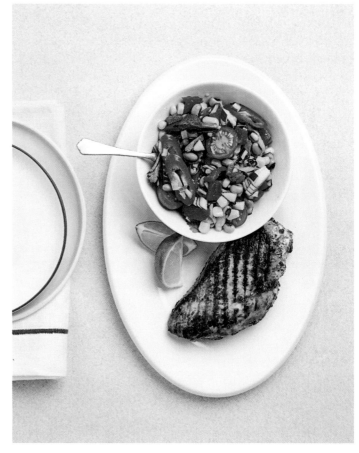

Place the chicken in a sandwich bag or non-metallic bowl with the tomato purée, chipotle paste and lime zest and season to taste. Close (or cover) and leave to marinate in the fridge for 30 minutes or overnight if you want to get ahead. Sometimes, if I'm really pushed for time, I leave out the marinating time.

Heat the oil in a nonstick griddle pan and pop in the chicken. Griddle, turning occasionally, until beautifully stripy on both sides and cooked through – about 10 minutes in total.

Meanwhile, mix all the salsa ingredients in a large bowl and season to taste. Serve with the griddled chicken, with lime wedges to squeeze over.

# WATERMELON 'STEAK' SALAD ⓥ

This salad is just perfection when you want to impress – and it tastes like summer. This dish is lighter on protein than most, so you can add a portion of griddled chicken or have it alongside any of the burgers (see pages 179, 198 and 206).

SERVES 2

1 mini watermelon
50g (½ cup) pitted black olives
100g (scant 1 cup) cherry tomatoes, quartered
70g (2½oz) rocket
70g (2½oz) goats' cheese, crumbled
1 tablespoon chopped toasted hazelnuts

FOR THE DRESSING
1 tablespoon aged balsamic vinegar
1 tablespoon extra virgin olive oil
1 teaspoon wholegrain mustard
sea salt and black pepper

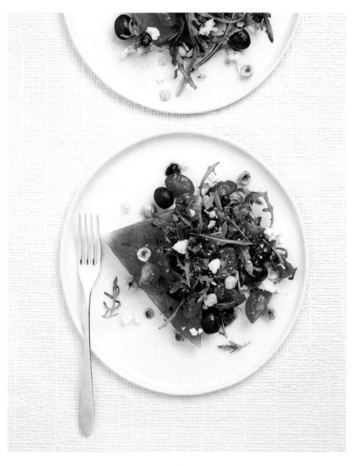

Cut two chunky circular slices from the middle of the melon, slicing right the way through. Keep the rest of the melon for a smoothie or fruit salad. Cut around the slices with a small knife, removing all the skin and any white parts. Now poke out the seeds. Arrange the 2 watermelon 'steaks' on plates.

Mix the dressing ingredients in a small bowl and set aside. Gently toss together the olives, cherry tomatoes, rocket and goats' cheese and pile on top of the watermelon.

Scatter over the hazelnuts and drizzle with the dressing before serving.

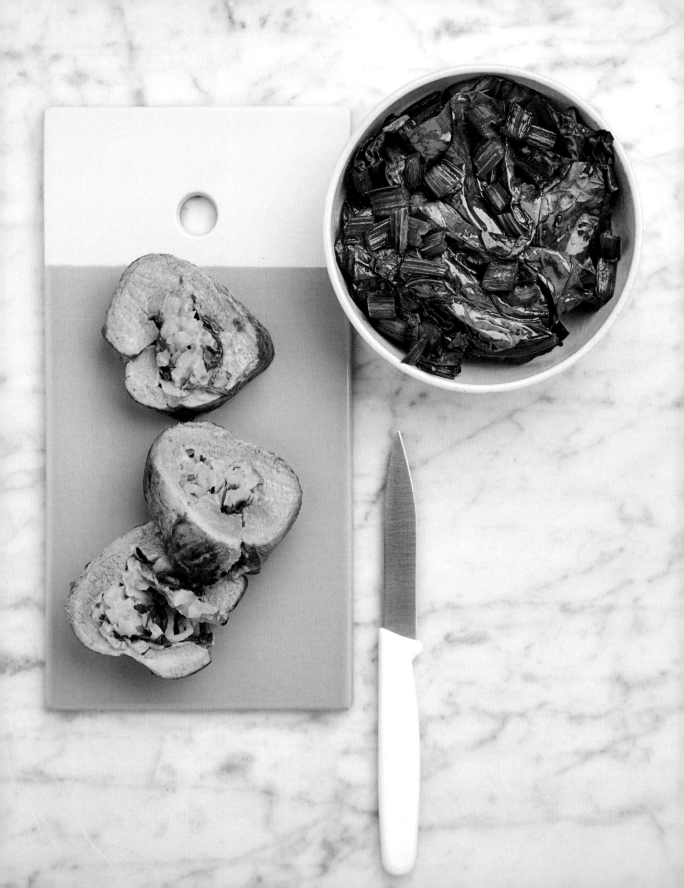

# STUFFED PORK FILLET WITH RAINBOW CHARD

This is one of my favourite Sunday lunches. The lean pork fillet is kept so moist with the infusion of flavours in this easy stuffing. Anchovies season the chard beautifully, but you can season with sea salt flakes if you're not a fan.

2 tablespoons olive oil
1 fennel bulb, cored and finely sliced
1 large leek, finely sliced
2 garlic cloves, crushed
finely grated zest of 1 lemon
50g (1¾oz) rocket, chopped
450g (1lb) piece of pork fillet
1 tablespoon Dijon mustard
sea salt and black pepper

## FOR THE CHARD
small knob of unsalted butter
2 marinated anchovy fillets from a jar
or can, chopped
400g (14oz) rainbow chard, stalks and leaves
chopped separately
finely grated zest and juice of ½ orange

Preheat the oven to 220°C/425°F/Gas Mark 7.

Heat the oil in a large frying pan over low-medium heat and cook the fennel and leek until they are completely softened and lightly caramelized. Stir in the garlic, lemon zest and rocket and season to taste. Take off the heat and set aside.

Next prepare the pork. Lay the pork on a board and make a horizontal cut into the side of the fillet, right along its length. Stop cutting just before you reach the opposite edge of the pork, so the two pieces remain attached. Open out the fillet like a book, then make further cuts into the fillet along its length to flatten it out as much as you can. Next use a rolling pin to bash it out to a more even thickness.

Spread the mustard over the pork, then press on the leek mixture. Roll up the pork from one of the long sides and secure in place with a few pieces of kitchen string.

Give the frying pan a wipe, then return to the heat. Carefully brown the pork fillet, turning until golden on all sides. Transfer to a baking sheet and cook in the oven for 25 minutes or until cooked through. Cover with foil and leave to rest while you cook the chard.

Heat a large frying pan over a medium heat and add the butter and anchovies. Fry the chard stalks for a few minutes until nearly cooked, then add the orange zest and juice and chard leaves. Cook until wilted. Slice the pork, removing the string as you go, and serve with the chard.

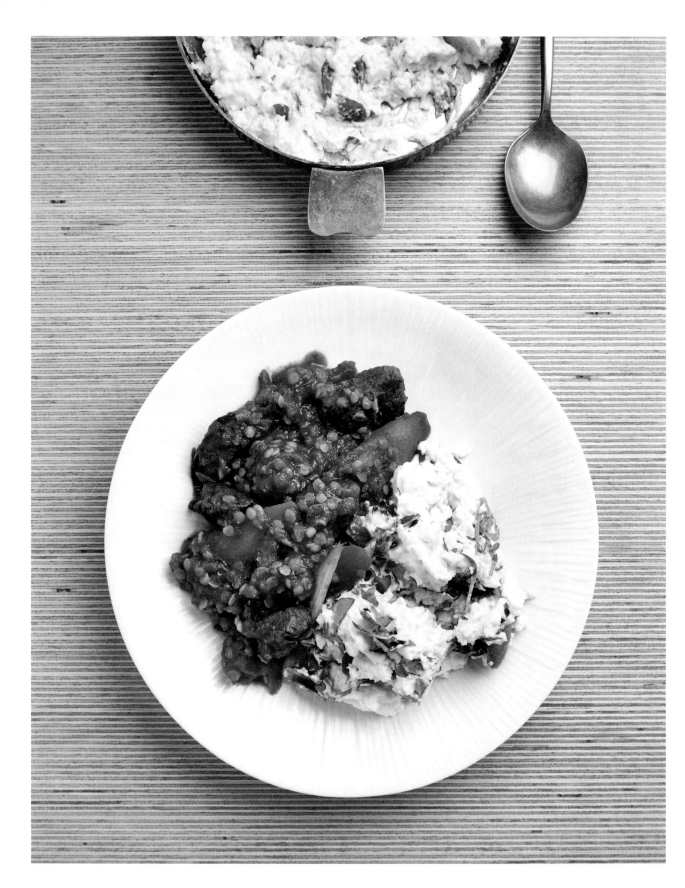

# BRIDGEN BEEF STEW

This might look like a lot of ingredients, but it's so simple to make and the slow cooking does all the work. You can make the stew ahead and freeze it, so this recipe is great for batch-cooking. Cauliflower mash is a wonderful potato substitute, and is so good at soaking up all the delicious stew juices.

1 tablespoon vegetable oil
1 large red onion, chopped
2 carrots, chopped
3 celery sticks, chopped
500g (1lb 2oz) lean braising steak, diced
3 tablespoons tomato purée
800ml (3¼ cups) good beef stock
2 x 400g (14oz) cans chopped tomatoes
1 rosemary sprig
1 thyme sprig
½ teaspoon fine salt
½ teaspoon black pepper
100g (½ cup) dried red lentils,
rinsed in cold water

FOR THE CAULIFLOWER MASH
1 large cauliflower, cut into florets
(about 700g/1lb 9oz)
1½ tablespoons hot horseradish sauce
50g (scant ¼ cup) low-fat cream cheese
50g (1¾oz) watercress, chopped
sea salt and black pepper

Heat the oil in a large saucepan over medium heat and cook the onion, carrots and celery until starting to soften. Turn up the heat a bit, add the steak and cook, stirring, until browned all over.

Stir in the tomato purée, 500ml (2 cups) of the stock, the canned tomatoes, herbs, salt and pepper. Bring to the boil then simmer gently for 1½ hours until the beef is nearly tender, skimming off any surface fat as the beef cooks.

Add the lentils to the stew and the remaining stock if the stew looks dry. Simmer for 20 minutes more until the lentils are tender.

For the cauliflower mash, cook the cauliflower florets in a saucepan of salted boiling water for 5 minutes. Drain well and allow to steam dry for a few minutes (otherwise the mash might be soggy).

Return the cauliflower to the pan with the horseradish and cream cheese and mash well. Season the mash, have a taste and add a little more horseradish if you like. Mix through the chopped watercress and serve the mash with the stew.

# INDEX

# ACKNOWLEDGEMENTS

It takes a village of people to get a book to print, and I've a huge number of people to thank for their support over the last few months.

There would be no books at all without my agent, Heather Holden-Brown aka 'Matron', whose steely determination for the book's success gave me the confidence to try my hand at writing. I thank you hugely for always telling me what I need to hear, when I need to hear it and for your great friendship.

I owe the deepest gratitude to my Editorial Director, Eleanor Maxfield. You are an amazing woman, and I thank you deeply for the success of all the Louise Parker Method books. You are a dear friend to me and I owe you a spa break or maybe a 28-day programme in Arizona for your patience and motivation over the last few months. Four years ago, Eleanor was 'Chief Cheerleader' to commission my first book. Then, along with Team Octopus, got me tiddly to celebrate hitting *The Sunday Times* Bestseller List with book one, and *The Cookbook* was commissioned. Another *Sunday Times* Bestseller and I thought I'd been rather lucky and should quit while ahead. But on a flight home from LA last summer, I felt kind of empty that I had not written a book that summer. The first email on landing was Eleanor asking for a meeting. The seductive – and exceptional – team at Octopus won me over for book three. And here we are. Thanks for your incredible faith in me, even when I was unable to see it for myself.

The entire team at Octopus, Hachette are exceptional, passionate and I admire you all hugely. Managing Director, Denise Bates, who I have the greatest respect for, Kevin Hawkins (the best Sales Director), Pauline Bache, who edits all my recipes and words until it all pulls together into a proper book, and Caroline Alberti, the Production Controller who makes sure everything prints perfectly. I admire your patience and thank you immensely for working with me on such a tight timeline. And last but not least, the utterly brilliant Art Director, Yasia Williams-Leedham, who has been like a wise, calm sister to me throughout, and whose creative eye makes these beautiful picture books such a treat. Thank you for your constant encouragement throughout. Without you and Eleanor, I'd honestly not have made it to deadline – the juggle just felt so hard.

But you working mums inspired me to just break it down a week at a time. I thank you both deeply for not giving up on me when others might have.

These beautiful pages are a collaboration of so many talents. Photographer, Chris Terry has shot all the Lifestyle and cover pics for all my books. I just love working with you Chris, you're absolutely brilliant and laughing so damn hard throughout, helps to put me at ease. Always an absolute blast and joy to work with you. Thank you big time my friend. Huge thanks to the splendid talent of Louise Hagger, who has photographed my recipes so beautifully so many times and really made the recipes come to life. They really are such a treat, Lou, thank you darling. And the divine Natalie Thompson, Food Stylist extraordinaire, who has styled all my recipes – which includes cooking hundreds of them exactly as per recipe (letting me know when I've been haphazard with an ingredient so tactfully) and presenting them in such beautiful way. Stylist, Alexander Breeze, created such beautiful scenes to make each food shot pop. Thank you all, it's always such an honour and huge fun to work with you.

I owe so much to my friends who have cheered, pushed and kindly lied about my talents on days I needed motivating, to get me to the finish line. I have learned it takes very dear friends to be so understanding of my absence on so many occasions I'd have loved to be at these last few months. You know who you are. I never fear hard work, but not being fully present for friends and family is a hard feeling to bear. There aren't enough words to give sufficient thanks to all my friends for their understanding. I'd like to give special thanks to Lucy Clarke, Louise Button, Sian Davies, Daniel Meltzer, Sharon and Jess Ridler, Dr Dambisa Moyo, Jenny Papenfus, Anna Boss, Stephanie Rix, Jessica Callan, Deirdre Stewart and Federika Brant.

There were long weeks where I was absent from my husband Paul and my daughters. Yet they all just kept cheering me on. My daughters would not allow me to quit. 'You can do it, Mummy' chanted Sophie daily, forgiving me softly for my absence. And Milly's daily mantra 'Dream Big, Don't Give Up' kept me inspired. Dear Chloe didn't seem to worry as long as I'd return home with treats and tight hugs, always reciprocated deeply. I wonder if it hadn't been for my daughters, I'd have postponed this book until an easier time. I'm so delighted they kept me going and we know now that there's nothing we can't finish that we put our minds to it, when we have loving support. I could burst with pride for my daughters – Sophie, Milly and Chloe. They really are my greatest pride, purpose, joy and inspiration.

I think, if you have a chance, you must always take it. Ride the wave of every opportunity while it is there. My dear friend Federika taught me this and I hope to pass this lesson on to my girls. They are so proud of what goes on behind the 'Orange Door' (our wellness company, Louise Parker) and take such interest in every member of our lovely team. They took delight in spending Sundays in our clinics with Paul, as I curled up on the sofa with a blanket, tea and laptop. I'd arrive at work jaded on a Monday with inspirational quotes on my desk. I've kept them all.

My work family are beyond exceptional and their unwavering loyalty and enthusiasm have meant so very much to me. How we have evolved over the last few years and I have never been prouder of the team that we are today. Thank you for your passion for all that we do and your consistent striving to help others. There is not enough space to list all your individual names and talents, but you know who you are. I thank you all from the bottom of my heart for all that you give to make our unit as tight and progressive as can be. I thank all our dieticans, personal trainers and our exceptional operations team at Walton Street and Harrods. My Lead Dieticians, Alejandra McCall RD and Reshma Patel RD run a tight, professional, loving team and I thank you in particular for your support and friendship. Special thanks to personal trainer, Robyn McEvoy, based in our Harrods studios, for training with me and helping me to change up the workouts for the purpose of this book. You stepped in and helped when my mind hit a blank and reminded me not to overcomplicate things. You are such a joy and working with you is an honour.

And Emma Holyoake, my assistant of seven years – there are no words. Thank you dear Em for your unwavering support and kindness. You know I could not do any of it without you and you really are the most special friend to me.

I have the greatest respect for my entire team at Louise Parker – thank you all. You're all bloody brilliant and to work with you all is such a privilege. I am so excited to work with you on our upcoming projects and developing the Method and work that we do. How I lucked out with a team of such kind, intelligent and loyal pros fills me with gratitude. It's taken some bumps and lessons – all of which make us tighter and stronger.

Special thanks go to all our clients at Louise Parker, the readers and followers of my first two books – who are an astonishingly supportive and loving Tribe. The Insta Tribe #leanietribe and #louiseparkermethod kept me determined to finish with your constant support. I'd have felt I'd let you down had I not made it, and so huge thanks to each and every one of you. Helping you helps me, more than you know. Your passion for the Method and the community you have formed is humbling. You're phenomenal and I'm so proud of all the friendships that we have formed.

Life has dealt my family a tough card this year. It has not been an easy time. I missed days – and I can't share the details as they are not mine to share – that I will always regret deeply. It has come at great cost and there were so many days I honestly felt I should postpone this book to be with my family. Mummy in particular encouraged me to crack on, and so I did. The courage, understanding and love that runs so deeply through our family has made me even more thankful for you all. How lucky we are really. I know that once this book is out, we will be celebrating a new year together, in good health. Thank you to all the Maynards, Parkers and Dollars. I am so blessed to have such a beautiful family.

My deepest love and gratitude goes to my husband Paul. His devotion, passion, humour and family values sustain and nurture us all, through the best and worst of times. I'm so proud of the life we have built together, with the support of an astonishingly loving extended family and friends. Everything we have been blessed enough to hold dear, is because of you. And when it all feels too much, you've taught me never to give up, find the lesson and joy and always crack on, no matter what. I love you beyond words.

An Hachette UK Company
www.hachette.co.uk

First published in Great Britain in 2018 by Mitchell Beazley,
an imprint of
Octopus Publishing Group Ltd
Carmelite House
50 Victoria Embankment
London EC4Y 0DZ
www.octopusbooks.co.uk

Distributed in the US by
Hachette Book Group
1290 Avenue of the Americas
4th and 5th Floors
New York, NY 10104

Distributed in Canada by
Canadian Manda Group
664 Annette St.
Toronto, Ontario, Canada M6S 2C8

ISBN 978-1-78472-537-2

A CIP catalogue record for this book is available from the
British Library.

Printed and bound in China

10 9 8 7 6 5 4 3 2 1

Publisher's Acknowledgements
**Editorial Director** Eleanor Maxfield
**Art Director** Yasia Williams-Leedham
**Senior Editor** Pauline Bache
**Copy Editor** Jo Smith
**Designer** Abi Read
**Photographers** Louise Hagger and Chris Terry
**Illustrator** Lizzy Thomas
**Food Stylist** Natalie Thomson
**Prop Stylist** Alexander Breeze
**Hair & Make-up** Victoria Barnes
**Production Manager** Caroline Alberti
With thanks to Laain for supplying sportswear for this book.
For more details, please visit laain.co.uk